Praise for
MIND Over MED

"The revised edition of Dr. Lissa Rankin's groundbreaking work, Mind Over Medicine, goes even deeper into how our emotions and traumas can contribute to disease, and her new 6 Steps to Healing Yourself are a glorious guide for anyone looking to jump-start their healing, whether it be physical, emotional, spiritual, or all of the above."

— **Kelly A. Turner, Ph.D.**, New York Times best-selling author of
Radical Remission and Radical Hope

"In this updated edition of an original gem, Dr. Lissa Rankin joins the hard-earned wisdom of her own healing journey with the science of mind/body unity. Doing so, she gifts us with a primer on the impact of personal transformation on physiological health and a unique guide to achieving mental and physical well-being."

— **Gabor Maté, M.D.**, author of When the Body Says No: Exploring the Stress/Disease Connection

"This revised edition of Mind Over Medicine takes a fresh look at the research informing the original classic that has been the go-to book for so many people who have been awakening to their capacity to take unprecedented control of their health, well-being, and destiny."

— **Jeffrey Rediger, M.D., M.Div.**, Harvard Medicine School faculty,
author of CURED: The Life-Changing Science of Spontaneous Healing

"As a physician, teacher, and writer, I'd like to recommend this book to ALL of my patients! Dr. Rankin summarizes, with simple and descriptive detail, how anyone can engage the most powerful healer of all—their own body."

— **Rachel Carlton Abrams, M.D., M.H.S., ABoIM**, author of BodyWise:
Discovering Your Body's Intelligence for Lifelong Health and Healing

"Lissa Rankin's Mind Over Medicine is a gift to us all. Lissa's clarity, compassion, and truth-telling wisdom shine throughout this book and take us on a journey out of victimhood into science-based healing empowerment. If you're ready to open to the magic of your healing journey, read this book."

— **Dr. Shamini Jain**, founder and CEO, Consciousness and Healing Initiative;
Assistant Professor, University of California, San Diego

"Lissa Rankin is a true scientist in the sense that she follows the data even though it challenges some of what she wrote in her best-selling first edition of this book. In this new edition, her delightfully personal and engaging writing style brings to life her journey of discovery regarding not only the mind's power to heal . . . but also the fact that there are parts of many people that fear or aren't ready for healing. The inclusion of a step addressing this constraint makes her program comprehensive and fully effective. It's a beautiful and important book!"

— **Richard Schwartz, Ph.D.**, creator of the Internal Family Systems model of psychotherapy

"What a pleasure it is to see the next generation of physicians waking up to what I call real medicine—the kind that acknowledges our true power to heal and be well."

— **Christiane Northrup, M.D.**, OB/GYN physician and author of the New York Times bestsellers Women's Bodies, Women's Wisdom and The Wisdom of Menopause

"Lissa Rankin is a modern-day miracle worker with a message the world needs to hear."
— **Chris Guillebeau**, *New York Times* best-selling author of *The $100 Startup*

"In her life, her work, and her words, Dr. Rankin demonstrates a new way to combine the brilliance of modern science with the wisdom of the heart. . . . Just reading Mind Over Medicine is a genuinely healing experience."
— **Martha Beck, Ph.D.**, author of *Finding Your Way in a Wild New World*

"Being my own inner physician for years means that I'm SUPER thrilled about Dr. Lissa Rankin's brilliant new book, Mind Over Medicine. . . . Lissa's writing style is so exuberant and deep at the same time, it makes me feel like I can do handstands on the ocean!"
— **SARK**, author of 16 books, artist, and founder of PlanetSARK.com

"Mind Over Medicine *modernizes age old messages of wisdom and makes them easier to understand and apply to modern day lifestyles. This book contains much wisdom in easy-to-apply lessons we can all learn from.*"
— **Bernie Siegel, M.D.**, author of *Love, Medicine & Miracles*

"With humor, warmth, and compelling research, Dr. Lissa Rankin's Mind Over Medicine *begins to heal the most critical fracture of our time—the break between our mind, bodies, and spirit.*"
— **Brené Brown, Ph.D.**, *New York Times* best-selling author of *Daring Greatly: How the Courage to Be Vulnerable Transforms the Way We Live, Love, Parent, and Lead*

"This is a compelling, clear, and reader-friendly vision of where medicine and healing are headed, written by an expert medical insider who's been there. Buy two copies—one for you and one for your doctor."
— **Larry Dossey, M.D.**, author of *Reinventing Medicine, Healing Words*, and *One Mind*

"WOW! Just wow! That is how I feel about Lissa Rankin's work! Everything she says rings so true to me, and her voice, as a professional medical doctor, is just what is needed in today's drug dependent society. Bravo, Lissa for having the courage to speak out and share your truth. This world needs more like you!"
— **Anita Moorjani**, *New York Times* best-selling author of *Dying to Be Me*

"An M.D. herself, Rankin takes on the establishment from the inside out, building a compelling argument for a new approach to health and healing that puts the patient in the driver's seat. Prepare to have your mind blown . . . and your body healed."
— **Jonathan Fields**, author of *Uncertainty* and founder of the Good Life Project

"Lissa Rankin sheds scientific and mystical light on our ability to self-heal. She is a doctor for those of us who know in our bones that vitality is ours for the making."
— **Danielle LaPorte**, author of *The Fire Starter Sessions*

"Mind Over Medicine *is one of the most comprehensive and compassionate guides for healing that I have come across. Dr. Rankin blends evidence-based research with the more psychosocial elements of love, community, and belief in an empowering and hopeful recipe for true holistic healing.*"
— **Kelly Noonan Gores**, writer/director/producer, *Heal* documentary

MIND
over
MEDICINE

ALSO BY LISSA RANKIN, M.D.

The Fear Cure*

The Anatomy of a Calling

The Daily Flame

What's Up Down There?

Encaustic Art

*Available from Hay House
Please visit:

Hay House USA: www.hayhouse.com®
Hay House Australia: www.hayhouse.com.au
Hay House UK: www.hayhouse.co.uk
Hay House India: www.hayhouse.co.in

LISSA RANKIN, M.D.

MIND
over
MEDICINE

Scientific Proof That
You Can Heal Yourself

REVISED EDITION

HAY HOUSE, INC.
Carlsbad, California • New York City
London • Sydney • New Delhi

Copyright © 2013 by Lissa Rankin
Revised Copyright © 2020

Published in the United States by: Hay House, Inc.: www.hayhouse.com®
Published in Australia by: Hay House Australia Pty. Ltd.: www.hayhouse.com.au
Published in the United Kingdom by: Hay House UK, Ltd.: www.hayhouse.co.uk
Published in India by: Hay House Publishers India: www.hayhouse.co.in

Cover design: Julie Davison • *Interior design:* Nick C. Welch

All rights reserved. No part of this book may be reproduced by any mechanical, photographic, or electronic process, or in the form of a phonographic recording; nor may it be stored in a retrieval system, transmitted, or otherwise be copied for public or private use—other than for "fair use" as brief quotations embodied in articles and reviews—without prior written permission of the publisher.

The author of this book does not dispense medical advice or prescribe the use of any technique as a form of treatment for physical, emotional, or medical problems without the advice of a physician, either directly or indirectly. The intent of the author is only to offer information of a general nature to help you in your quest for emotional, physical, and spiritual well-being. In the event you use any of the information in this book for yourself, the author and the publisher assume no responsibility for your actions.

The Library of Congress has cataloged the previous edition as follows:

Rankin, Lissa, 1969-
    Mind over medicine : scientific proof you can heal yourself / Lissa Rankin, M.D. -- 1st edition.
        pages cm
    ISBN 978-1-4019-3998-4 (hardback) -- ISBN 978-1-4019-4000-3 (digital)
1. Mental healing. 2. Spiritual healing. 3. Mind and body therapies. I. Title.
        RZ400.R15 2013
    615.8'528--dc23

                                                                    2012048461

Tradepaper ISBN: 978-1-4019-5988-3

13 12 11 10 9 8 7 6 5

1st edition, May 2013
2nd edition, June 2020

Printed in the United States of America

In loving memory of David,
my beloved Daddy,
the original Dr. Rankin

CONTENTS

PREFACE TO THE REVISED EDITION

Natural forces within us are the true healers of disease.

— HIPPOCRATES

Back in 2009, when I first dove down the rabbit hole of the science of spontaneous remissions and the placebo effect—a journey that would result in the phenomenon that became *Mind Over Medicine*, including several TEDx talks; two national public television specials; the Whole Health Medicine Institute, a consciousness and healing training program for health-care providers; and Heal At Last, a community of people practicing the Six Steps to Healing Yourself together—I was blessedly naïve about how deep down the rabbit hole I would be called to travel. Although mind-body medicine has been in the zeitgeist for at least half a century, I was not raised by open-minded hippie parents and was not exposed to mind-body practices at home or in medical school. It was not until I left my job as a conventionally trained physician working in a hospital in 2007 that I was first introduced to best-selling books that had been published in my lifetime and gobbled up by the public, such as *Love, Medicine & Miracles*, by Bernie Siegel, M.D.; *The Relaxation Response*, by Herbert Benson, M.D.; *Minding the Body, Mending the Mind*, by Joan Borysenko, Ph.D.; or *Kitchen Table Wisdom*, written by the doctor who would become my mentor, Rachel Naomi Remen, M.D. On the contrary, I was raised by a rigidly skeptical physician father and a family full of Methodist ministers and missionaries, where I was brought up to separate science and spirituality at all costs. Any attempt to combine the two was judged as New Age nonsense or charlatanism at best—or the work of the devil at worst. This kind of childhood programming set me up to be the least likely person on the planet to write a book like this.

Had I known what I would discover on this journey to where science and spirituality intersect, I might have spun around on my heels and hightailed it in the opposite direction. But curiosity combined with cluelessness led me down the rabbit hole. As Rachel Naomi Remen, M.D., told me, "Sometimes the soul grabs you by whatever handle is sticking out and leads you back home to yourself." Back in 2009, the handle that was sticking out was my rabid fascination and insatiable inquisitiveness about the mysterious healings my patients seemed to be experiencing when I was not ordering special laboratory tests, giving them prescription medication or supplements, or treating them with surgery. I didn't understand how people who had been sick with chronic diseases and life-threatening illnesses were experiencing unexplained cures and crediting them to whatever medicine I seemed to be offering. Back then, I didn't understand how powerful an effect deep inquiry, loving presence, and a safe, sacred space for healing could have. I also hadn't cultivated the humble respect I now have for the human body's miraculous capacity to heal itself under the right conditions and with the right loving support.

Since this book was first published in 2013, a lot has changed in my life and in my consciousness, as well as in science and the world at large. As part of my research for the book I'm working on as this revised edition goes to press—*Sacred Medicine: A Doctor's Quest to Unravel the Mysteries of Miraculous Healing*—I spent nearly a decade studying with shamans in Peru, qigong masters from China, Balinese healers, Hawaiian kahunas, gurus from Eastern religious traditions, indigenous medicine men and women, biofield scientists and physicists from around the world, and energy healers, trauma therapists, and faith healers from my own country. I visited sacred sites reputed to facilitate healing, such as Lourdes and the Santuario de Chimayó, where people report experiencing mysterious, unexplainable healings. Because the handle sticking out back then dragged me around the globe in search of answers, I now have the opportunity to come back to the research that lies at the root of *Mind Over Medicine* with a fresh yet grounded perspective, informing this revised edition of the book that has become a classic for people who are on a healing journey from illness, injury, or trauma.

Letting Go of Control

Like most doctors, I am a bit of a control freak. Although I didn't realize it consciously at the time, the conditions of my childhood and a need to feel safe left me yearning to control life and death, as many doctors seek to do. Surely, if I were armed with the best education on the planet, protected from uncertainty with scientific knowledge and medical skills, then I could master the insecurities inevitable to life in a human body, right? Ha! How little I understood back then. Fortunately, most foibles coexist with a silver lining. This unconscious desire to control life and death birthed what you are about to read in this book. Since patients of mine were experiencing what my friend, cancer researcher Kelly Turner, Ph.D., calls "radical remissions," I wanted to hack the healing process so I could add new understanding to the body of knowledge I learned in medical school. I feel tender for the parts of me that so desperately wanted to control life back then, for those parts fueled my passionate quest to learn what I share with you here.

Even the title of this book reflects my own state of consciousness when I first wrote it. "Mind Over Medicine" suggests that the all-powerful mind can control your reality, and all you have to do is learn to harness it. I desperately wanted that to be true. If it was, then I could comfortably hold on to my old-world view: that doctors are in control of life and death, only now we need to help patients control the mind, in addition to practicing good medicine. The possibility that we might *not* be capable of controlling life and death was just too distressing to me at the time I first wrote this book. Now I'm more comfortable with the unknown and more willing to trust the mystery rather than trying to control life. I think of the book more as "Consciousness Over Medicine" or maybe even "Consciousness IS Medicine." I no longer believe that healing is a purely mental process, but I do believe that expanding your consciousness has the potential to cure life-threatening diseases and shift your whole life, and this book will help you do that.

With age comes wisdom, and as I work on the revised edition of this book, I am just now integrating the tensions inherent in the paradoxical nature of reality. Ten years ago, I would have said, "You can heal yourself," and I realize now this is half true. It's true that taking charge of your health can move you out of the disease-inducing frequency of victimhood and transition you into the health-inducing state of realizing that you can impact your reality with the brave lifestyle choices you have the power to make. It's also true that most people can't heal themselves alone. Some people take "self-help" too far and stress their nervous systems with the all-American story of the rugged individualist, with the idea that you can make anything happen if only you push and strive and exert the power of your will hard enough. I now find it more true to hold the paradox of doing what you can to be proactive about healing yourself while simultaneously surrendering to the flow of an unknowable Mystery so vast that we cannot fathom it with our cute little pea brains. Such seeming contradictions run rampant when you go as far down the rabbit hole of researching healing as I've gone.

Since writing the first edition, I've also witnessed far too many people in the New Age world exaggerating claims about healing and preying upon vulnerable sick people who are desperate to end their suffering or extend their lives. This may be a smart marketing ploy, but it's not fully honest. The truth is that we participate in the creation of our reality, and this book is intended to help you be proactive about doing what you can to participate in your healing, but it is naïve to believe you control life, death, or healing. Tied into the patterns of control that dominate our culture is our fear of death, even our demonization of it. Yet death is part of life. The birth of every new moment is the death of the last. I want to make sure nobody ever interprets my body of work to mean that if you *don't* heal, you are a spiritual failure. Nothing could be further from what I intend here.

So What's New in This Revised Edition?

In part, you'll learn why I now teach the Six Steps to Healing Yourself in a different order, with two steps collapsed into one and one additional, critical step, which I'd missed the first time around, tacked onto the end. It took me years of teaching *Mind Over Medicine* workshops to realize that I had had several blind spots when I wrote the first edition. These simple but potent modifications can significantly impact the efficacy of the Six Steps. For many years, I've been teaching the Six Steps to Healing Yourself differently when I teach doctors and healers in the Whole Health Medicine Institute how to facilitate this process in patients, but my updated modifications were only available to those in my professional training programs. Now, dear reader, you'll learn the revised sequence of healing steps, as well as my rationale for making these changes.

I'm also updating some of the scientific references, since science moves fast and we are learning at an unprecedented rate as science undergoes its own revolution, fueled by maverick scientists who refuse to dogmatically dig their heels into scientific materialism in the face of new scientific discoveries that upend what we thought we knew about the nature of reality.

You'll also be introduced to the elephant in the room that never got clearly identified in the original edition, namely that as long as there's unhealed trauma in your body's system, complete cure from chronic and life-threatening illnesses may elude you, and when cure does happen, it may not be permanent. This doesn't mean you have to have experienced the big "T" traumas, such as childhood sexual abuse or addiction in the family or going to war, in order for healing trauma to be relevant to potentially curing illness permanently. We have all endured what Buddhist psychiatrist Mark Epstein, M.D., calls "the trauma of everyday life"—the situational and developmental traumas that keep us from living in alignment with our purest essence, or what I call your "Inner Pilot Light," which you'll read more about in the pages ahead. When we are denying what is not working in our lives, pushing ourselves to conform to a society on the brink of environmental devastation and moral collapse, suppressing our emotions, suffering in silence by ourselves, living in social isolation, ignoring our intuitions, disconnecting from our spiritual lives, or otherwise turning away from the truth of our deepest knowing, our nervous systems instinctively react as if a predator is out to get us, triggering the biochemistry of "fight or flight," which disables the body's natural self-healing abilities. Yet many of us are doing this unwittingly, thinking we are doing what we must to live a healthy lifestyle, not realizing that with trauma reverberating in our systems we are creating in our bodies the perfect setup for disease.

This is nobody's fault. As Indian philosopher Jiddu Krishnamurti said, "It is no measure of health to be well adjusted to a profoundly sick society." So why are we pathologizing people who are depressed, anxious, and sick in the presence of a sick culture? When sensitive people feel sad, angry, frustrated, helpless, hopeless, and in pain, why are we diagnosing them with mental or physical disorders rather than acknowledging that their empathic response to the state of affairs in the world is, in fact, a normal, healthy reaction to the kind of dehumanizing behavior many others have simply become numb to? Wouldn't we be better off devoting ourselves to healing our culture rather than medicating what's normal and stigmatizing, drugging, or hospitalizing those who have tender hearts and energetic sensitivity? Why not turn the billions of dollars we spend on pharmaceuticals toward activism aimed at restoring the sacred in the world?

Don't get me wrong. As you'll see if you read this book carefully, I never have been and never will be "anti–Western medicine." I'm eternally grateful for medical technology and fully supportive of using it wisely, but not indiscriminately. I'm just making the case that no one can be blamed for succumbing to the conditioning our society programs into us. It is no wonder so many are sick and medicated, given how far off the rails our culture has led us. Yet once we know we have other ways of living, being, and healing, we have the potential to shift our relationship with disease and wellness, expanding our consciousness to include not only the miracles of Western medicine but also the untapped potential of the body-mind-spirit connection.

Although this approach to healing may not be for everyone, what I can say after nearly a decade of feedback from people who have felt moved to include the science, teachings, and practices of what you'll read in this book in their own Prescriptions for optimal health is that, should you say YES to the call from within that asks you to embark upon this kind of healing journey, your life will never be the same. You are the caterpillar entering the chrysalis, unlikely to come out of the cocoon unchanged. You may feel like you're dissolving in the process, the way the caterpillar becomes bug soup first rather than just sprouting wings as a butterfly. You will question everything and enter willingly or not so willingly into a place of uncertainty. This might feel unsettling, frightening even, as your ideas about yourself and perhaps even your worldview begin unraveling. You enter what Charles Eisenstein calls "the space between stories," when one story has ended but another story has not yet emerged.

In that space, you will find your Inner Pilot Light; and in the divinity you will discover within your humanity, healing happens; and with healing, cure sometimes follows. If this leaves you unsettled, let me reassure you by saying that if you can trust the journey and even borrow faith from the hundreds of thousands of people who have embarked upon this journey before you, you will discover that you have within you everything you need to be all that you must be. Dare I say that you will become the embodiment of what your soul came here to planet Earth to become? Sometimes this will result in full and permanent cure, and you will feel like you've been blessed with a miracle. Sometimes it will not, and I won't be able to explain why, but I do know that it's probably not because you failed to do something right.

Whatever the outcome, what I can promise you is that the potent inquiries likely to arise from within you as a result of this book will both challenge and illuminate you. The access to synchronicity and intuition that may open is likely to surprise and delight you. The heart-opening that accompanies these practices, which serve as what cardiologist and mind-body pioneer Dean Ornish, M.D., calls "a conspiracy of love," will help facilitate the longest journey you'll ever make—the journey from the head to the heart. By relaxing your mind with the science you will read in these pages, you open a portal that makes a life led by the heart but wisely informed by the intellect more available. All together, these transformations are likely to make your body ripe for miracles. Keep in mind that there is no way to do this right or wrong. As Mary Oliver writes in her poem "Wild Geese," "You do not have to be good. / You do not have to walk on your knees / for a hundred miles through the desert, repenting. / You only have to let the soft animal of your body / love what it loves." In other words, *relax*. Do what you can, but don't overdo it. The healing that is possible may be right here, closer than close, underneath all your efforting and striving, available if you are ready to humble yourself before this possibility and receive what awaits you.

INTRODUCTION

There is no illness of the body apart from the mind.

— SOCRATES

What if I told you that caring for your body is the *least* important part of your health . . . that for you to be truly vital, other factors are more important? What if the key to health isn't just eating a nutritious diet, exercising daily, maintaining a healthy weight, getting eight hours of sleep, taking your vitamins, balancing your hormones, or seeing your doctor for regular checkups?

Certainly, these are all important, even critical, factors to optimizing your health. But what if something else is even more important?

What if you have the power to heal your body just by changing how your mind thinks, your heart feels, and your life force flows?

I know it sounds radical, especially coming from a doctor. Trust me, I was just as skeptical when I first discovered the scientific research suggesting that this might be true. Surely, I thought, the health of the human body isn't as simple as thinking ourselves well or worrying ourselves sick.

Or is it?

After 12 years of conventional medical education and 8 years of clinical practice, I had been thoroughly indoctrinated into the dogmatic principles of evidence-based medicine, which I worshipped like the Bible. I refused to trust anything I couldn't prove with a randomized, controlled clinical trial. Plus, having been raised by my father, a very conventional physician who made fun of anything New Age, I was as hard-nosed, closed-minded, and cynical as they come.

The medicine I had been trained to practice didn't support the idea that you can think yourself well or make yourself sick with the power of your thoughts and emotions. Sure, my medical school professors diagnosed some illnesses that lacked biochemical explanations as "all in the patient's head," but those patients were promptly and quietly referred to psychiatrists, while eyes were rolled and heads were shaken.

It's no wonder the notion that the mind might have the power to heal the body would be threatening to many mainstream doctors. After all, we spend a decade learning the tools that supposedly give us mastery over other people's bodies. We want to believe that the time, money, and energy we've put into becoming doctors isn't wasted. We're professionally and emotionally invested in the idea that if something breaks down physically, you must seek our expertise. As doctors, we like to believe we know your body better than you do. The whole medical establishment is based on such a notion.

Most people are happy to function within this paradigm. The alternative—that you have more power to heal your own body than you've ever imagined—lobs the responsibility for health back into your court, and many people feel like that's just too much responsibility. It's much easier to hand over your power and hope some expert who is smarter, wiser, and more experienced can "fix" you.

But what if we've got it all wrong? What if, by denying the fact that the body is naturally wired to heal itself and the mind impacts this self-healing system, we're actually sabotaging ourselves?

As physicians, we inevitably see things happen on our watch that science simply can't explain. Even the most closed-minded doctors witness patients who get well when, by every scientific rationale, they shouldn't. When we witness such things, we can't help questioning everything we hold dear in modern medicine. We start to wonder if there is something more mystical at play.

Doctors don't usually discuss this possibility in front of patients, but they do whisper about it in the doctors' lounges of hospitals and inside conference rooms at Ivy League universities. If you're curious and you pay attention—like I do—you hear stories, stories that blow your mind.

You hear people whispering about the woman whose cancer shrank away to nothingness during radiation. Only afterward did the doctors discover that the radiation machine was busted. She hadn't actually received one lick of radiation, *but she believed she had*. So did her doctors.

They talk about the woman who had a heart attack followed by bypass surgery, then wound up in shock, which led to full-blown renal failure, believed to be fatal without treatment. When the doctors offered dialysis, she refused treatment, not wanting to endure more invasive procedures. For nine days, her kidneys made no urine, but on the tenth day, she started peeing. Two weeks later, with no treatment, she was back to working out, and her kidney function was better than before her surgery.

Then there's the man who had a heart attack and refused heart surgery only to have his "incurably" blocked coronary arteries open up after changing his diet, beginning an exercise program, doing yoga, meditating daily, and attending group therapy sessions.

Another patient who was hospitalized in the ICU and whose organs were shutting down from stage 4 lymphoma had a near-death experience, became one with pure, unconditional love, and instantly knew that if she chose not to cross over to the other side, her cancer would disappear almost at once. Less than a month later, her lymph nodes were biopsied, and no evidence of cancer remained.

Yet another woman broke her neck. After being taken to a hospital and getting X-rays that confirmed that she had broken her neck in two places, she opted to refuse medical intervention and saw a faith healer instead, despite her doctors' vehement objections. Without any medical treatment, she was out jogging a month later.

One story floating around claims that a research protocol for a chemotherapy drug called EPOH was getting some marginally positive results, but one oncologist was demonstrating wildly successful outcomes. Why? Rumor has it he switched around the name of the drug protocol when he discussed it with patients. Instead of injecting his patients with EPOH, he injected them with HOPE.

Then I read the *New York Times* article[1] about the Greek war veteran who was sent to the United States in the 1940s for treatment of a combat-mangled arm. He got work doing manual labor in the U.S., married a Greek American woman, and settled down to have children. When he noticed that he was getting short of breath while doing his work, he went to the doctor and was diagnosed with terminal lung cancer and told he had only nine months to live. He was offered aggressive treatment, but after nine months doctors apparently assured him that it wouldn't save his life, he decided to save his money, decline treatment, and move with his wife back to his native Ikaria, a Greek island, where he could be buried with his ancestors in a graveyard overlooking the Aegean Sea.

He and his wife moved with his elderly parents into a small house on a vineyard, where he expected he would die soon. While he prepared to die, he reconnected with his faith and started going to his old church. When his friends got wind of the fact that their old buddy was back home, they showed up with bottles of wine, books, and board games to entertain him and keep him company. He even planted vegetables in a garden, not expecting he'd be around to harvest them. Over the next few months, he basked in sunshine, savored the salty air, and relished in his love for his wife.

Six months passed, and not only did he not die; he was actually feeling better than ever. He started working in the untended vineyard during the day, making himself useful, and in the evenings, he'd play dominoes with friends. To get to church, he had to climb up and down the hills of Ikaria, which, over time, he was better able to manage. Every day, he, like many other residents of Ikaria, drank a homemade herbal tea sweetened with honey, which is believed by the locals to cure all that ails you. He took a lot of naps, rarely looked at a watch, and spent a lot of time outdoors.

Forty-five years later, the man who'd allegedly had end-stage cancer celebrated his 98th birthday. He never underwent treatment. At one point, 25 years after his diagnosis, bewildered by what had happened, he went back to the United States to ask his doctors for an explanation. In an ironic twist of fate, the doctors who had treated him were all dead.

Then there's the young nurse practitioner whose sarcoidosis led to end-stage heart failure, who didn't qualify for a heart transplant because her destructive disease would likely destroy her new heart. Her doctors told her to get her affairs in order because she had only three to five years to live. They underestimated her body. A year later, she came barreling up to me with a copy of her latest echocardiogram. Her doctors couldn't believe her heart had healed itself and she now had perfectly normal function.

As I heard these stories, I couldn't ignore the gnawing voice within me. Surely, these people couldn't all be liars. But if they weren't lying, the only explanation was something *beyond* what I had learned in conventional medicine.

It got me thinking. We know spontaneous, unexplainable remissions sometimes happen. Every doctor has witnessed them. We just shrug our shoulders and go on about our business, usually accompanied by a dull, unnerving sense of dissatisfaction because we can't explain the remission with logic.

But in the back of my mind, I've always pondered whether it's possible we have any control over this process. If the "impossible" happens to one person, is there anything we can learn from what that person did? Are there similarities among the patients who get lucky? Are there ways to optimize the chances of spontaneous remission, especially when effective treatment doesn't exist in the standard medical toolbox? And what, if anything, can patients or doctors do to facilitate this process?

I couldn't help wondering if, perhaps, by not at least *considering* the possibility that patients might have some control over healing themselves, I was being an irresponsible doctor and violating the sacred Hippocratic oath. Surely, if I were a good doctor, I would be willing to open my mind in service to the patients I cared for.

But inspiring stories bandied about in doctors' lounges or floating around on the Internet simply weren't enough to convince me. A scientist by training and a skeptic by nature, I needed cold, hard proof, and when I started asking for it, I came up short.

I did my best to investigate the rumors I was hearing. I started asking the people telling me their stories to prove them. Could they show me slides under the microscope? Could I talk to the mechanic responsible for the radiation machine? Could I see the medical records?

I was mostly disappointed. When I asked for medical records or studies as backup, most people apologized. "It was so long ago."

"There was definitely a study, but I don't have the reference." "My doctor retired, so I can't put you in touch." "They threw away my medical records."

Even the instances of self-healing I vaguely remembered witnessing in the earlier days of my own practice were out of my reach. I hadn't kept notes. I couldn't remember names. I didn't know how to contact these people. I kept hitting dead ends.

Yet the more questions I asked online, the more stories kept flowing in. When I started getting nosy with my physician friends, every doctor I asked told me jaw-dropping stories of unexplained spontaneous healings, patients who wound up cured from "incurable" illnesses, leaving those who pronounced them "terminal" looking like fools. But still, they had no proof.

By this point, I was intrigued, bordering on obsessed. My curiosity led me to dig deeper. After hundreds of e-mails and dozens of interviews, I came to believe that something real was happening to these patients whose stories became lore in metaphysical books and on the Internet. Although it's tempting to dismiss the often ridiculous-sounding stories of patients who claim to have healed themselves, if you're a doctor who cares about helping others heal, you can't ignore what you hear. The more you listen, the more you start to wonder just what the body is capable of.

Most doctors, if you get them away from their often critical and judgmental colleagues, will admit this: deep down, they believe that when it comes to the healing process, some crossover between the mystical and the physiological is at play, and that the common ground that connects the two seems to be the great and powerful mind, as well as what you might call the spirit or the soul. But few say so out loud for fear of being labeled quacks.

The mind-body-spirit link has been advocated by medical pioneers for decades. Yet, in spite of this, it has failed to shoulder its way into the mainstream medical community. As a young doctor, I received my medical degree well after renowned physicians such as Bernie Siegel, Christiane Northrup, Larry Dossey, Rachel Naomi Remen, and Deepak Chopra had raised awareness about the mind-body-spirit link, and you might think their teachings would have been included as part of my medical education. But I was largely unfamiliar with their work until long after I finished medical school. Not until I began doing my own research did I even read their books.

Once I finally did, I was pissed. How had I not known who these open-minded, open-hearted doctors were? And why were their books not required reading for medical students and first-year residents?

As I learned more, I got all riled up, and that passion turned into a mission that fueled several years' worth of research and writing. I started reading every mind-body-spirit medicine book I could find. I also started blogging, tweeting, and posting on Facebook about what I was learning, which only increased the frequency with which I heard stories from people who had experienced what can only be described as medical miracles. I was riveted. The evidence was mounting. But nothing I was hearing counted as "science." I craved scientific proof that it wasn't total nonsense.

So I kept researching, willing my mind to stay open as I learned more about how the mind could affect the body. Part of me was open to the whole mind-body-spirit concept. It made intuitive sense to me. But another part of me was wildly resistant. To believe what I was learning would require letting go of much of what I had been taught, both from my very traditional physician father and from my medical school teachers.

One of the first books I studied, Harvard professor Anne Harrington's mind-body medicine history book, *The Cure Within*, left me feeling physically dizzy and viscerally unsettled. In the book, she refers to the mind-body phenomenon as "bodies behaving badly," meaning that sometimes bodies don't respond the way they "should," and the only way we can explain such mysteries is through the power of the mind.[2]

As examples of bodies behaving badly, Harrington tells stories of children living in institutional settings whose material needs were all met but who wound up developmentally and mentally stunted because they were improperly loved. She also cites 200 cases of blindness in a group of Cambodian women forced by the Khmer Rouge to witness the torture and slaughter of their loved ones. Although medical examination could find nothing wrong with the eyes of these women, they claimed to have "cried until they could not see."[3]

Clearly, something was up. The butterflies in my belly drove me to dig deeper, and as I did, I became fascinated with understanding how these things had happened. What proof did we have that the power of the mind could transform the body? What physiological forces could explain such occurrences? And what might we do to harness these healing powers?

If I could answer these questions, I could begin to make sense, not just of the mind-boggling stories people were telling me, but of the purpose of my own life and my role as a healer.

At the time I was researching the mind-body-spirit link, my place in the world of medicine was unclear to me. For many years as a physician, I had operated under a false assumption. I had spent 12 years training to become a doctor, ostensibly so that I would know more about the bodies of my patients than they did. Doctors are body experts, right? I was trained that patients come to doctors because they are broken and, supposedly, we know how to "fix" them.

Growing up with a physician father, I thought only doctors cured sick people. It wasn't even on my radar to think that patients could potentially heal themselves and that, as a result, radical remission without medical intervention might be in the realm of possibility. As a medical student and resident, I believed it was my responsibility to diagnose what was wrong with a person's body and prescribe the right treatment. If they got better, I credited myself. If they didn't, I blamed myself.

As a practicing physician, I felt the weight of my job—to make the right assessments, settle on the right diagnoses, and deliver the proper treatments without ever making a mistake. Aside from hoping my patients would participate in lifestyle modifications like smoking cessation, exercise, and a better diet, I didn't expect much of them. I certainly didn't expect them to heal their own bodies. That's what I was there for.

But after I became more experienced as a young doctor, I had a sneaking suspicion I might have it all wrong. After all, who knows the patient's body better than the patient? While doctors may know the names of the arteries in the hand or the muscles in the leg better than most patients, in some cases, especially those related to stress, the patient is actually the best diagnostician. Perhaps, instead of believing we doctors know what's best for the body, patients would be better off diagnosing the root causes of their illnesses and writing their own Prescriptions for what needs to change in their lives in order to make their bodies ripe for miracles. After all, that's what I ended up doing on my own healing journey as a patient.

My Healing Journey

By the time I was 33 years old, I was stressed out, burned out, and living in a near-constant state of fear, anxiety, and overwhelm. I was extremely unhappy in my job as a full-time partner in a busy obstetrics and gynecology practice, where I was expected to work 36- or 72-hour shifts in the hospital, performing surgeries and delivering babies. I had become disillusioned with our broken healthcare system, which required me to churn through 40 patients a day, often scheduled in hurried seven-and-a-half-minute slots, leaving little time for us to actually talk, much less bond. My heart felt broken when a longtime patient wrote to tell me she had planned to confess to a sensitive health issue she was hiding from me. She had rehearsed what she would say for days, with the support of her husband. But when it came time for her to spill the beans, she wrote, I never removed my hand from the exam-room door. My hair was disheveled and I was dressed in dirty scrubs. She suspected I had been up all night delivering babies—and I probably had been. Although she knew I was probably tired, she kept praying I would touch her arm, sit down on the stool next to her, and offer enough tenderness and connection to make her feel safe to talk about her concern.

But, she said, my eyes were blank and I never let go of the door handle.

When I read that letter, I got choked up, felt a hiccup in my chest, and knew in my heart that practicing this kind of medicine was not what drew me to my profession. I had been called to medicine the way some are called to the priesthood, not to churn out prescriptions and blow through physical exams like a machine but to be a healer. What drew me to the practice of medicine was the desire to touch hearts, to hold hands, to offer comfort amid suffering, to enable recovery when possible, and to alleviate loneliness and despair when cure wasn't possible. If I lost that, I would love everything.

Every day of being a doctor was chipping away at my integrity. I didn't have language for it at the time, but Harvard doctors are now calling it "moral injury,"[4] the same kind of traumatic wound that war veterans experience when they follow orders that require them to betray their own ethics. It was eroding my mental, physical, and spiritual health to practice medicine inside a corrupt system that gives lip service to patient well-being but, in practice, prioritizes the financial bottom line. I knew the kind of medicine my soul wanted to practice, yet I felt helpless to reclaim the doctor-patient connection I craved, as well as victimized by managed-care companies, the pharmaceutical industry, malpractice lawyers, politicians, and other factors that threatened to widen the rift between me and my patients. But what were my alternatives? I was the sole breadwinner in my family, responsible for covering my medical school debt, my husband's graduate school debt, the mortgage, and my newborn daughter's college fund. Quitting my job was out of the question.

On top of my stressful job, I was also twice divorced, I had lost several people I loved to cancer, and I was feeling profoundly lonely and depressed. Basically, my stress responses were firing off all day long, and it should have come as no surprise that my body was breaking down.

Years earlier, in my 20s, I had been diagnosed with multiple health conditions, including high blood pressure; cardiac arrhythmias; a painful sexual disorder called vulvar vestibulitis; severe, debilitating allergies; and precancerous changes on my cervix. I took seven medications, got weekly allergy shots, and underwent surgery on my cervix. But in spite of all the drugs and procedures, my blood pressure was still out of control, my allergies were so bad I could barely leave the house, I couldn't have sex without feeling like I was getting stabbed with a knife, my heartbeat was skipping around like a Mexican jumping bean, and my cervix still showed precancerous changes, even after surgery.

In short, I was a hot mess on my way to an early heart attack or cervical cancer, and my doctors didn't know what to do with me.

I wound up falling head over heels for the man who would become the father of my daughter, Siena. My health improved to some degree after falling in love. But I was still loading up on drugs every day, and my body was far from well. While I was pregnant with my daughter, my father was diagnosed first with prostate cancer, which was treated, and then six months later with melanoma metastatic to the brain and liver. This news, in addition to some cracks in the armor that allowed me to participate in an increasingly corrupt health-care system, led me to a suicidal breakdown when I was 24 weeks pregnant. While I could override the moral objection my childhood religion had ingrained in me toward taking my own life, I couldn't bring myself to take my baby's. My ability to force function through the integrity breaches inherent to my job was crumbling.

You could say that Siena saved my life. I wound up giving birth to my daughter by C-section, and a few days later, when I should have been in a postpartum glow of bonding and love with my newborn, my healthy young brother wound up in full-blown liver failure as a rare side effect of the antibiotic Zithromax, which he was taking for a sinus infection. He was told he'd likely need a liver transplant, which further eroded my faith in the conventional medical system I had trusted so fully my whole life. Then my beloved dog died just before my father passed away, exactly two weeks after I had given birth. I was devastated by the crisis I came to call my "Perfect Storm."

Just when I was coming up for air, my partner, Matt, who was the full-time caregiver for our newborn, cut two fingers all the way off with a table saw. Although the surgeon was miraculously able to replant them with medical technology, Matt was unable to care for our daughter, Siena, for months. All hell broke loose in our lives.

With my stress responses on overdrive, it's no surprise my body, as well as my mental state, began to downslide again. I was nearly paralyzed from the emotional and physical pain I experienced, and suicide was rarely far from my mind. I wound up feeling like I was squished from all sides, succumbing to pressures I couldn't control that pushed me deeper and deeper down into a dark place, as though I were stuck in the narrows of a birth canal, barely able to breathe.

But there was a bright side. The traumas I experienced during my Perfect Storm put a rip in the mask I had been wearing to fit in and get by. When that rip shredded the mirage of my seemingly perfect life, I came to discover a long-lost part of myself I now call my Inner Pilot Light.

That's when I knew that somehow, some way, I would survive this ordeal. But it wasn't going to be easy.

Facing the life changes I knew I needed to make, I was terrified. Examining the truth about my life was like standing on the edge of a neck-breaking cliff and staring down into the vast unknown. I had a newborn baby, a temporarily disabled and unemployed husband, a sick brother, a widowed mother who was grieving, a mortgage, graduate school debt, and no backup plan. With no safety net, I left medicine, planning never to look back. Selling the house, liquidating my retirement account, and downsizing, moving my family to the country to live a simple life, I chalked the whole doctor thing up to one big, fat mistake and planned to be a full-time artist and writer. People ask me now how I was brave enough to quit my job, but I never saw it as brave. I saw it as saving my life. When the pain of staying put exceeds the fear of the unknown, you leap. That terrifying leap initiated my journey to healing.

Now, mind you, healing yourself is not for the faint of heart. It's also not something you can do with the force of your will. At first, I tried to just grab myself by the ovaries and make some scary-ass choices, but bullying myself didn't work. The only thing I could do, over and over again, was surrender, often in tears, to the force of love that had created me and trust that if there was something I was meant to do, my Inner Pilot Light would show me the way. (For a guided meditation that helps you practice this kind of surrender, sign up for the Connect to Your Inner Pilot Light program at Inner PilotLight.com.)

I spent two years growing increasingly deeper in debt while I hiked every day, practiced yoga, learned to meditate, participated in transformational workshops, got into therapy, spent a lot of time in Big Sur at Esalen Institute, painted in my art studio, found my spiritual mentor in *Kitchen Table Wisdom* author Rachel Naomi Remen, M.D., and started writing my first book. But something didn't feel right, and I started feeling a painful longing in my heart. The truth was that, as much as I was enjoying painting and writing, I missed my patients.

I didn't know when I left the hospital that you can quit your job, but you can't quit your calling. I couldn't imagine going back to the hospital. I sensed it might kill me. But I realized I needed to find a way to express the healer inside me. When I was offered a job at an integrative medicine practice in Marin County, near San Francisco, it felt like kismet. In West Marin County, I'd have the chance to live by the ocean, where the redwoods meet the mountains, right off scenic Highway 1. The environment felt like medicine, and the doctors I would be practicing with were open-minded and interested in alternative methods of healing.

I had a hard time envisioning a way to practice medicine that would allow me to live in alignment with my values, but the lovely physician in charge of the integrative medicine practice offered me the world—as much time as I wanted with my patients, the opportunity to use the beautiful, healing space to lead workshops, an invitation to showcase my art, and free rein to create a sacred practice aligned with my healer heart. I lit up like a Christmas tree and jumped at the chance.

On-the-Job Training

I was not prepared for the way this job would threaten my still very conventional worldview. When I joined the new practice, I was in awe of my new patients. They were the most health-conscious people I've ever had the privilege to serve. Many who came to the center drank their daily green juice, ate a vegan diet, worked out with personal trainers, slept eight hours a night, took a handful of vitamins and other health supplements every morning, spent a fortune on seeing complementary and alternative medicine (CAM) healers, and religiously followed the orders of the best doctors from UCSF and Stanford. This regimen worked wonders for some. They were pinnacles of health with glowing skin and gorgeous bodies and life force emanating through their pores.

But others were some of the sickest people I'd ever cared for in my life. I was baffled! I had worked with patients in the inner city of Chicago and Somali refugees on the Mexico–United States border. With their poverty, lack of access to healthy lifestyles, limited medical care, and extensive trauma histories, I understood why they were sick. But these Marin County patients were some of the sickest people I'd ever cared for in my life! It made no sense based on how I had been trained to understand health. From everything I had learned in medical school, these people should have been in perfect health. So why were so many "healthy" patients suffering?

In my attempts to help these patients, I ran batteries of tests, including specialized functional medicine tests conventional doctors don't usually order, and occasionally I'd pick up something surprising that, when treated, resulted in complete resolution of the patient's symptoms. The patients with whom that happened thought I was a superhero. One simple hormone replacement, for example, would transform their lives.

But with the subset of patients who lived healthy lives and still experienced boatloads of symptoms—more often than not, I'd find nothing and wind up shrugging my shoulders. I couldn't find a biochemical explanation for why these patients didn't feel vital. I felt like a failure, but I sensed in my heart it wasn't my fault. I wasn't forgetting to order some critical test. I hadn't failed to refer them to the right specialist. The answer resided elsewhere. There was still a big missing piece of the healing puzzle behind all these mystery illnesses. I just couldn't figure out what it was.

By this time I was really curious and motivated to solve the puzzle of why these "healthy" patients were so sick. Instead of focusing exclusively on health behaviors, past medical history, and other traditional questions, I started asking my patients to tell me about their lives. Because we had the luxury of an hour to spend together, I could sit and listen. And what they started telling me changed how I viewed the whole notion of health.

That's when I got inspired to change my patient intake form. Instead of limiting my questions to the patient's past medical history, past surgical history, family history, medications, and history of substance use, the way I had been taught to do in medical school,

I added a laundry list of questions to my intake form about the rest of the patient's life. What I learned from these questions amazed me.

A Radical New Kind of Patient Intake

I started digging deep into the personal lives of my patients, asking questions most doctors had never thought of: Is anything keeping you from being the most authentic, vital *you*? If so, what is holding you back? What do you love and celebrate about yourself? What's missing from your life? What do you appreciate about your life? Are you in a romantic relationship? If so, are you happy? If not, do you wish you were?

Are you fulfilled at work? Do you feel like you're in touch with your life purpose? Do you feel sexually satisfied, either with a partner or by yourself? Do you express yourself creatively? If so, how? If not, do you feel creatively thwarted, like there's something within you dying to come out? Do you feel financially healthy, or is money a stressor in your life?

If your fairy godmother could change one thing about your life, what would you wish for? What rules do you follow that you wish you could break?

I also started taking an extensive trauma history on my patients, and I found that the people with the fattest charts often had the longest, most painful trauma histories. When I asked whether they had seen therapists, many said, "Yes, but it didn't help, so I don't go anymore."

I discovered that my patients' answers often gave me more insight into why they might be sick than any lab test, medical record review, or X-ray exam could. The diagnosis was often crystal clear in a way I had previously missed because I wasn't asking the right questions.

I came to see that these patients were unhealthy, not because of bad genes or poor health habits or rotten luck, but because they were gut-wrenchingly lonely or miserable in their bad relationships, stressed about work, freaked out about their finances, profoundly depressed, or suffering from a huge load of unhealed trauma. Most, when I asked on my intake form "What's missing from your life?" wrote a long list. And when I asked the same question in person, the majority of these patients wept. Something was going on that had nothing to do with vegetables or exercise or vitamins.

On the flip side, I had other patients who ate poorly, exercised rarely, forgot to take their supplements, and enjoyed seemingly perfect health. When I read their intake forms, they revealed that their lives were filled with love, fun, meaningful work, financial abundance, creative expression, sexual pleasure, spiritual connection, and other traits that differentiated them from the sick health enthusiasts. They also tended to report less trauma, or they admitted to having done a lot of psychological or spiritual inner work that they felt had helped them clear much of their trauma burden. They were, in essence, happy and fulfilled. And even though they didn't take the best care of their bodies, their bodies responded with good health.

That's when I began asking my patients two mother-lode questions: "What do you think might lie at the root of your illness?" and most important, "What does your body need in order to heal?" I now also ask the question Rachel Carlton Abrams, M.D., asks in her book *Bodywise*: "What would it take to live a life your body would love?"

When I first started popping these questions, I assumed people would tell me that the root cause of their illness was a hormone imbalance or an unhealthy diet. I thought they might share treatment intuitions with me. Things like "I think I'll choose craniosacral therapy over physical therapy" or "I'm gonna wait on that cholesterol drug and try changing my diet instead."

Occasionally, patients answered with insights into conventional health-related modifications they felt they needed to make—things like "I really need an antidepressant" or "Antibiotics should do the trick" or "I need to lose 20 pounds" or "I really need to get my hormones balanced."

But more often than not, when I asked, "What do you think might lie at the root of your illness?" my patients said things like these: "I give until I'm depleted." "I'm miserable in my marriage." "I absolutely hate my job." "I need more 'me' time." "I'm so lonely I cry myself to sleep every night." "I'm out of touch with my life purpose." "I don't feel God anymore." "I hate myself so much I can't look at myself in the mirror." "I'm avoiding facing the truth." "I can't forgive myself for what I've done." "I'm living a lie and I feel like a total fraud."

And when I asked my patients, "What does your body need in order to heal?" my patients shocked me with their answers: "I have to quit my job." "It's time to finally come out of the closet to my parents." "I must divorce my spouse." "I have to finish my novel." "I need to hire a nanny." "I'm so lonely; I need to make more friends." "I need to meditate every day." "I have to tell my husband I'm having an affair." "I need to stop being such a pessimist." "I need to forgive myself." "I need to love myself."

Whoa . . .

While many patients simply weren't ready to do what their intuition was telling them their bodies needed, the patients who were ready for real transformation listened to the quiet voice within and made radical changes. Some quit their jobs. Some finally committed to doing the deep trauma–clearing therapeutic work that actually releases trauma from the body. Others left their marriages. Some moved to new cities. Others finally pursued long-suppressed dreams.

The results these patients achieved were astonishing. Sometimes, a laundry list of illnesses would disappear, often very quickly. My patients were healing themselves after years of medical therapies had proven useless. I was in awe.

My Radical Remission

Living in Marin County led me further down my own healing path. I met with spiritual counselors, started drinking loads of green juice, cleared more trauma through a variety of therapeutic relationships and practices, explored my erotic self, devoted myself to a spiritual path that incorporated earth-based and embodiment-based spiritual practices, and climbed mountains daily. In 2009, I began blogging about what I missed about medicine, what I loved about medicine, what originally drew me to the practice of medicine, and what I was learning in my integrative medicine practice. I wrote about how I consider medicine a spiritual practice, how you *practice* medicine, the way you practice yoga or meditation, like you'll never fully master it. I wrote about how the doctor-patient relationship, when treated with the awe it deserves, is sacred, and how I longed to reclaim it. I wrote about how medicine had wounded me and how, in turn, I had inadvertently wounded others.

Patients and healers of all types started writing me e-mails, telling me their stories, posting comments on my blog, and something in me lit up, something that felt like an opportunity to be of service. The circle of people I attracted started healing *me*.

I had frequent dreams of sitting at the bedsides of patients from the past, the ones I hadn't had the time to fully attend to. In the dreams, I listened to their stories with no eye on my watch and no hand on the door. I'd wake up in tears, as if I had retrieved a piece of my soul. My new practice allowed me to heal what had been broken in me. With a whole hour to spend with patients, I was finally able to open my heart, listen, and practice true healing arts.

Around this time is when those remarkable stories of patients who healed themselves from *incurable* and *terminal* illnesses started trickling in, not just from the patients in my practice but from people all over the world. I didn't understand what was happening to my patients. They were crediting me with their cures, but I hadn't done anything other than ask good questions and listen with love. It didn't make any sense to me, so I did what I always do when I don't understand something—I researched it.

I hadn't intended to become a researcher of radical remissions, but one serendipity after another led me down an unplanned, uncharted path, as if birds were dropping crumbs, blazing a trail to my Holy Grail. Books fell off the shelf. Physicians appeared on my path with messages for me. People in my online community sent me articles. Unbidden visions appeared like movies in my mind while I was hiking. Dreams appeared. Teachers called.

I started waking up from the deep anesthesia my medical education and years of practice had induced, and in my groggy haze, I began to see the light. One question led to another, and before I realized what was happening, I was knee-deep in journal articles, trying to ferret out the truth about what is happening in the body when the mind is healthy and why we get sick when the mind is unhealthy or when we become spiritually disconnected. I realized that I didn't have to order lab tests, prescribe drugs, or operate in order to be of service as a doctor. I could help even more people by discovering the truth about how to help people heal themselves. What followed was a deep dive into the gospels of modern medicine, the peer-reviewed medical literature, where I sought scientific proof that you can heal yourself in journals like the *New England Journal of Medicine* and the *Journal of the American Medical Association*. What I found changed my life forever, and my hope is that it will also change your life and the lives of your loved ones.

As I tried to wrap my confused mind around the phenomena I was observing with my patients who were experiencing radical remissions, I was finally able, with the help of my inner guidance, to reverse engineer what I was doing intuitively with patients into a process I came to call "The Six Steps to Healing Yourself," which I now teach to health-care providers in the Whole Health Medicine Institute and which you'll be learning how to practice on yourself and your clients in Part Three of this book.

All of these paradigm-shifting changes in my life translated into many transformations in my physical, emotional, mental, spiritual, and relational health. Through my local and online community, I discovered a tribe of people interested in consciousness who were committed to radical self-care and healing the world—the people I had been looking for my whole life. Suddenly, I was no longer lonely. I knew my life's purpose. I loved my work. My home environment was medicine for me. I was in love. I felt a deepening spiritual connection to all of life. And I was happier than I had ever been in my life.

One by one, I got off all of my medications and my health conditions completely resolved. Today, I'm off all of my allergy shots, my cervix has returned to normal without further surgery, my sexual disorder is gone, my cardiac arrhythmia has disappeared, and my blood pressure has normalized. As an added bonus, I lifted my mood from depressed to frequent bouts of joy, lightened my trauma load, bolstered my capacity for empathy and deep intimacy, deepened my connection to Source, and feel almost unbearably grateful to be able to do the sacred, transformational, creative, and activist work I do.

The Birth of *Mind Over Medicine*

This book dives deep into the journey of discovery I've just outlined and shares with you the scientific data I uncovered, which changed my whole outlook on how medicine should be delivered and received. Once I read this data, I knew I could never again pull the wool back over my eyes.

Is there scientific data to support the seemingly miraculous stories of self-healing that float around? You betcha. There's proof that you can radically alter your body's physiology just by changing your mind, opening your heart, and connecting to your spirituality. There's also proof that you can make yourself sick when your mind thinks unhealthy thoughts, your heart closes, and you're spiritually disconnected. And it's not just mental. It's physiological. How does it happen? Don't worry; I'll also explain exactly how unhealthy thoughts and feelings translate into disease and how healthy thoughts and feelings help the body repair itself.

But there's more. There's proof that doctors might facilitate your recovery, not so much because of the treatments they prescribe, but because of the authority you ascribe to them. There's also proof that one surprising factor can benefit your health more than eliminating cigarettes, that something you may consider unrelated to the health of the body can add more than seven years to your life, that one fun thing can dramatically reduce the number of doctor visits you'll need, that one positive shift in your mental attitude can make you live 10 years longer, that one work habit can increase your risk of dying, and that a pleasurable activity you probably never linked to a healthy life can dramatically reduce your risk of heart disease, stroke, and breast cancer.

These are just a few of the scientifically verifiable facts I share in this book that have radically changed how I think about medicine.

This book is divided into three parts. In Part One, I'll make the argument that the mind has the power to alter the body physiologically through a potent combination of positive belief and the nurturing care of the right health-care providers. In Part Two, I'll show you how the mind can alter the body's physiology based on the life choices you make, including the relationships you choose to nurture, your sex life, the work you do, your financial choices, how creative you are, how spiritually attuned you are, whether you live in a place your body loves, whether you're an optimist or a pessimist, how happy you are, and how you spend your leisure time. I'll also teach you one valuable tool you can use anywhere—one that could save your life.

All of this will set you up for Part Three, where I introduce you to a radical new wellness model I've created and guide you through the Six Steps to Healing Yourself, which have been revised and updated for this new edition of the book. For seven years, I've been training physicians and other health-care practitioners to facilitate patients through these six steps, but if you have even a good friend that can support you through the process, you can practice these six steps yourself and potentially benefit from the kinds of outcomes tens of thousands of people have reported as the result of doing this transformational healing work. By the time you finish the book, you'll have made your own diagnosis, written your own Prescription, and created a clear action plan designed to help you make your body ripe for miracles.

Keep in mind that the tips I give you aren't just for sick people but also for healthy people interested in preventing disease. I don't want you to wait until your body starts screaming at you with life-threatening diseases. Instead, I want to encourage you to listen to the whispers from your body: these are touchstones on your path to optimal health, leading you away from what predisposes you to illness and toward what has been scientifically proven to result in better health and vital longevity, setting you up to increase the likelihood that your health span will equal your life span.

What I'm about to reveal to you may surprise you—even, perhaps, threaten you. But please, do your body a favor, and as you read this book, try to withhold your judgments, open your mind, tune in to your heart and your intuition, and be willing to shift how you think about your body and your health. What I'm about to share with you may challenge long-held beliefs, knock you out of your comfort zone, and make you question whether I'm making this stuff up. But I swear I'm not. Throughout this book, I make every effort to back up what might seem like far-out statements with scientific references.

Because I know that what I'm about to teach you will raise eyebrows, I've written this book just for the people who are skeptical, as I was. I've laid out the book to walk you through my argument as if a jury of my physician peers were judging me. But it's not so much the doctors I'm aiming to convince. Sure, I hope they listen, because if they do, the face of modern medicine as we know it will change forever.

But really, I'm writing this book for *you*—for every person who has ever been sick or injured, anyone who has ever loved someone with an illness or disability, and anyone who wants to prevent illness. You're the one I yearn to help, because in my heart, I long to end suffering and help you optimize the chance that you will live a long, vital, healthy life. That mission is what called me to medicine in the first place.

As you read, I ask only that you stay with me. Give me a chance to expand your mind and touch your heart the way my mind and heart have been blown open. Let me help you expand your consciousness and heal your thoughts so your body can follow. And give yourself permission to release outdated notions about health and medicine. The future of medicine is upon us. Come, take my hand. Let's explore.

PART ONE

OPTIMIZE THE PLACEBO EFFECT

CHAPTER 1

THE SHOCKING TRUTH ABOUT YOUR HEALTH BELIEFS

What we are today comes from our thoughts of yesterday, and our present thoughts build our life of tomorrow: our life is the creation of our mind.

— THE DHAMMAPADA

A 1957 case study by Dr. Bruno Klopfer (who famously pioneered the Rorschach inkblot test) reports the story of Dr. Philip West and his patient Mr. Wright. Dr. West was treating Mr. Wright, who had an advanced cancer called lymphosarcoma. All treatments had failed, and time was running out. Mr. Wright's neck, chest, abdomen, armpits, and groin were filled with tumors the size of oranges, his spleen and liver were enlarged, and his cancer was causing his chest to fill up with two quarts of milky fluid every day, which had to be drained in order for him to breathe. Dr. West didn't expect him to last a week.

But Mr. Wright desperately wanted to live, and he hung his hope on a promising new drug called Krebiozen. He begged his doctor to treat him with the new drug, but the drug was only being offered in clinical trials to people who were believed to have at least three months left to live. Mr. Wright was too sick to qualify.

But Mr. Wright didn't give up. Knowing the drug existed and believing the drug would be his miracle cure, he pestered his doc until Dr. West reluctantly gave in and injected him with Krebiozen.

Dr. West performed the procedure on a Friday, but deep down, he didn't believe Mr. Wright would last the weekend.

To his utter shock, the following Monday, Dr. West found his patient walking around out of bed. According to Dr. Klopfer, Mr. Wright's "tumor masses had melted like snowballs on a hot stove" and were half their original size. Ten days after the first dose of Krebiozen, Mr. Wright left the hospital, apparently cancer free.

Mr. Wright was rockin' and rollin', praising Krebiozen as a miracle drug, for two months—until the scientific literature began reporting that Krebiozen didn't seem to be effective. Mr. Wright, who trusted what he read in the literature, fell into a deep depression, and his cancer came back.

This time, Dr. West, who genuinely wanted to help save his patient, decided to get sneaky. He told Mr. Wright that some of the initial supplies of the drug had deteriorated during shipping, making them less effective, but that he had scored a new batch of highly concentrated, ultra-pure Krebiozen, which he could give him. (Of course, this was a bald-faced lie.)

Dr. West then injected Mr. Wright with distilled water.

And a seemingly miraculous thing happened—*again*. The tumors melted away, the fluid in his chest disappeared, and Mr. Wright was feeling great again for another two months.

Then the American Medical Association blew it by announcing that a nationwide study of Krebiozen proved that the drug was utterly worthless. This time, Mr. Wright lost all faith in his treatment. His cancer came right back, and he died two days later.[1]

When I read this, I thought, *Yeah, right.* Surely, this case study couldn't be true. How could cancerous tumors just "melt like snowballs" in response to an injection of water? If the case report was true and something so simple could make a cancer go away, why weren't oncologists wandering through the wards, injecting stage 4 cancer patients with water? If they had nothing to lose, what was the harm?

The whole thing seemed improbable, so I kept looking. Surely, if there was any truth to such a story, there would be similar case studies reported in the literature.

Another patient reported in *The Journal of Clinical Investigation* suffered from severe nausea and vomiting. Instruments measured the contractions in her stomach, indicating a chaotic pattern that matched her diagnosis. Then she was offered a new, magical, extremely potent drug, which her doctors promised would undoubtedly cure her nausea.

Within a few minutes, her nausea vanished, and the instruments measured a normal pattern. But the doctors had lied. Instead of receiving a potent new drug, she had been dosed with ipecac, a substance known not to prevent nausea but to induce it.

When this nauseated patient believed her symptoms would resolve, her nausea and abnormal stomach contractions disappeared, even when the ipecac should have made them worse.[2]

I sat there scratching my head. Curious, but it didn't prove anything.

The Healing Power of Fake Surgery

Soon after, I stumbled across an article in the *New England Journal of Medicine* that featured Dr. Bruce Moseley, an orthopedic surgeon renowned for the surgeries he performed on people with debilitating knee pain. To prove how effective his knee surgery was, he designed a brilliantly controlled study.

The patients in one group of the study got Dr. Moseley's famous surgery. The other group of patients underwent an elaborately crafted sham surgery, during which the patient was sedated, three incisions were made in the same location as in the real surgery, and the patient was shown a prerecorded tape of someone else's surgery on the video monitor. Dr. Moseley even splashed water around to mimic the sound of the lavage procedure. Then he sewed the knee back up.

As expected, one-third of the patients getting the real surgery experienced resolution of their knee pain. But what really shocked the researchers was that those getting the sham surgery had the same result! In fact, at one point in the study, those who had received the sham surgery were actually having less knee pain than those who'd gotten the real surgery, probably because they hadn't undergone the trauma of the surgery.[3]

What did Dr. Moseley's patients think about the study results? As one World War II veteran who benefited from Dr. Moseley's placebo knee surgery said, "The surgery was two years ago and the knee has never bothered me since. It's just like my other knee now."[4]

This study hit me in the gut.

Mr. Wright and the lady getting ipecac were just case studies, and case studies, well known to have biases, aren't considered the gold standard when it comes to interpreting the medical literature. The gold standard by which I was taught to investigate scientific data is the randomized, double-blind, placebo-controlled clinical trial published in a peer-reviewed journal. Dr. Moseley's study, a randomized, double-blinded, placebo-controlled clinical trial—published in one of the most highly respected medical journals in the whole world—showed that a significant percentage of patients experienced resolution of their knee pain solely because they *believed* they had gotten surgery.

That was the first real evidence I collected that suggested to me that a belief—something that happens solely in the mind—could alleviate a real, concrete symptom in the body. Dr. Moseley's study is what led me to research the placebo effect, the mysterious, powerful, reliably reproducible treatment effect some patients experience when given fake treatment as part of a clinical trial.

The Powerful Placebo

Like every scientist, I had long known about the placebo effect. Fake treatments, such as sugar pills, saline injections, and sham surgeries, are routinely used in modern clinical trials to determine whether a particular drug, surgery, or treatment is truly effective. The term *placebo*, from the Latin for "I shall please," showed up in medical lingo ages ago to indicate inert treatments traditionally given to neurotic patients to placate them.

For centuries, doctors prescribed treatments without any clinical data to prove that the treatments themselves actually worked. Nobody questioned the treatments the doctor prescribed, and nobody did studies to prove whether something was effective. The doctors simply mixed up tonics, dosed up their patients, and the patients got better, at least a percentage of the time. Or the doctor cut someone open, performed a surgery, and the symptoms improved, or they didn't.

It wasn't until late in the 19th century that the idea of using placebos in clinical research began to emerge. Then, in 1955, the *Journal of the American Medical Association* published a seminal article by Dr. Henry Beecher called "The Powerful Placebo," which made the case that if you dosed people up with drugs, many got better. But if you gave them plain salt water or some other inert ingredient, about a third of them were also cured, not only in their minds, but in real, physiological ways that could be demonstrated in the body.[5]

Suddenly, the concept of "the placebo effect" became a mainstay of contemporary medicine, and modern clinical trials were born. Now good scientific studies bear the burden of proving that the healing effect of the drug or surgery being tested transcends the potent healing power of the placebo. If a drug or surgery demonstrates that it's more effective than a placebo, then it is deemed "effective." If not, the FDA probably won't approve the drug, the surgery will fall out of favor, and the treatment will be dismissed as ineffective, as Dr. Moseley's surgery was. Prescribing treatments that prove to be no better than a placebo is believed to violate the principles of evidence-based medicine. It's what separates the real doctors from the quacks.

Or so I was taught.

It got me thinking. What exactly is the placebo effect? Until I began my research, I had never really stopped to think about it. We all know people in clinical trials get better when you treat them with nothing but a sugar pill. But why?

That's when I realized I had hit the mother lode in my quest for proof that the mind can affect the body. If a percentage of people in clinical trials get better simply because they *believe* they're getting a real drug or surgery, the response they are getting is triggered *solely by the mind*. This realization threw me into a bit of a tailspin.

Evidence That Positive Belief Can
Alleviate Symptoms

Back to the medical journals I went, in search of more evidence that the mind's belief that the body is getting a drug or surgery is enough to result in real live symptom relief. I found that nearly half of asthma patients get symptom relief from a fake inhaler or sham acupuncture.[6] Approximately 40 percent of people with headaches get relief when given a placebo.[7] Half of people with colitis feel better after placebo treatment.[8] More than half of patients studied for ulcer pain have resolution of their pain when given a placebo.[9] Sham acupuncture cuts hot flashes almost in half (real acupuncture helps only a quarter of patients). As many as 40 percent of infertility patients get pregnant while taking placebo "fertility drugs."[10]

In fact, when compared to morphine, placebos are almost equally effective at treating pain.[11] And multiple studies demonstrate that almost all of the happy-making responses patients experience as a result of antidepressants can be attributed to the placebo effect.[12]

It's not just pills and injections that work wonders when it comes to symptom relief. As proven by Dr. Moseley's knee surgery study, sham surgeries can be even more effective. In the past, ligation of the internal mammary artery in the chest was considered standard treatment for angina. The thought was that, if you blocked blood flow through that artery, you'd shunt more blood to the heart and relieve the symptoms people experience when they're not getting enough coronary blood flow. Surgeons performed this procedure for decades, and almost all the patients experienced improvement in their symptoms.

But were they really responding to the ligation of the internal mammary artery? Or were their bodies responding to the belief that the surgery would be helpful?

On a quest to find out the answer, one study compared angina patients who got their internal mammary arteries ligated with patients who underwent a surgical procedure during which an incision was made on the chest wall, but the artery itself was not ligated.

What happened? Seventy-one percent of those subjected to the sham surgery got better, whereas only 67 percent of those who got the real surgery improved.[13] Internal mammary artery ligation now exists only in medical history.

The data I was collecting was impressive, and I had to wonder if it might be even more impressive if every effort weren't made to minimize the placebo effect in clinical trials. If researchers perceived the placebo effect as a positive phenomenon, something to embrace, perhaps we'd see even higher percentages. But that's not the focus most researchers have. On the contrary, clinical-trial coordinators and medical researchers (who are mostly employed by pharmaceutical companies) go out of their way to diminish the placebo effect. After all, patients who get better from placebos interfere with a drug's ability to get approved for market. To screen out those considered to have "excessive placebo responses," many randomized, double-blinded, placebo-controlled trials of drugs are actually preceded by a "washout phase," in which all participants take an inert pill and anyone who reacts favorably to it is eliminated from the study.

So, if the majority of researchers for new pharmaceuticals weren't getting paid handsomely by Big Pharma, we might see placebo response rates shoot even higher in clinical trials. I know this from personal experience, since I was once one of those clinical researchers, enrolling patients in pharmaceutical trials as a way to try to cover the skyrocketing cost of malpractice insurance and the overhead of running a practice in California, where reimbursement rates were plummeting. We were instructed by the pharmaceutical company to screen out the people who seemed to have an unusually exaggerated placebo response. In fact, after observing me with study patients, one pharmaceutical researcher suggested to me that I stop being so nice to my patients, since their symptoms seemed to be resolving before they even got randomized into the study. The goal of this research is to prove that the drug works better than placebo. If placebo rates are too high, it's hard to prove that a new drug is efficacious, since efficacy is defined as "better than placebo."

Does Everyone Respond to Placebos?

As I pondered the placebo effect, I found myself doubting whether I would ever respond to a placebo if I were a patient in a clinical trial. After all, I'm a doctor. I've been an investigator in clinical trials myself. I'm a smart cookie, and I think I'd just *know* whether I was getting a real treatment or not. If I suspected I was getting a placebo, clearly it wouldn't help me, right?

It got me thinking. Are certain types of patients more susceptible to placebo responses than others? Is there any data to suggest whether there's a classic profile for placebo responders? Are there personality traits or intelligence measures that predict who gets better when given a sugar pill? Do people with high IQs demonstrate less responsiveness to placebos? Are some people just more gullible?

Turns out scientists have studied this. Researchers originally postulated that those who responded to placebos would have lower IQs or be more "neurotic." But what they discovered is that nearly everybody can be induced to respond to a placebo under the right conditions. We are all susceptible, even doctors and scientists. In fact, some studies suggest that those with higher IQs are even more placebo responsive. Studies also found that optimists are more likely to respond to placebos than pessimists,[14] and that people who score higher for emotional resilience and friendliness respond more readily to placebos.[15] I took this as good news that it's not just gullible people who are vulnerable to placebo effects; it's also smarty-pants people like *you*.

Is Healing from Placebos All in Your Mind?

As my research continued, I couldn't quite wrap my brain around what I was learning. Clearly, the evidence I was collecting looked promising. When patients—not just the gullible ones but all patients—believe they might get well, a hearty percentage of them experience clinical improvement.

But this failed to fully satisfy my curiosity. I could make the argument that symptom relief really is all in your head. What is pain, after all, if not a perception in the mind? What is depression, if not a mental state? Even with more tangible diseases like asthma or colitis, maybe you just *perceive* that you can breathe better or *think* you have fewer gastrointestinal symptoms. Maybe the mental perception is changing, but the *body* isn't actually responding in any measurable physiological way. Maybe you just *think* it is, and that's enough to make you feel better.

If it's true that the mind can heal the body, there must be some way to demonstrate that the body is responding, not just with symptom relief, but in physiological ways that can be studied. The next phase of my research led me in search of proof that it's not all in your head, that the mind's belief can actually alter the body's physiology.

With hundreds of thousands of placebo-controlled trials published out there, finding an answer was no small feat, mostly because many of the studies I encountered evaluated symptoms such as headaches, back pain, depression, and decreased libido—which are difficult to quantify. When patients experience relief from such symptoms, it's largely subjective. There's no objective measurement that can prove that what they report is true.

But I did finally find proof that, at least a percentage of the time, real physiological changes happen in the body in response to placebos. When given placebos, bald men grow hair, blood pressure drops, warts disappear, ulcers heal, stomach acid levels decrease, colon inflammation decreases, cholesterol levels drop, jaw muscles relax and swelling goes down after dental procedures, brain dopamine levels increase in patients with Parkinson's disease, white blood cell activity increases, and the brains of people who experience pain relief light up on imaging studies.[16]

Five Traditional Explanations for the Placebo Effect

When clinical researchers talk about the placebo effect, they're actually referring to a whole host of events that happen when you bring people into a clinical setting, offer them a treatment that they know may be either the treatment under investigation or a placebo, and pay attention to them over a designated period of time. Let's clarify what those five explanations are so we're all using the right lingo.

The most obvious explanation is that patients experience symptom relief because they *expect* they will. Because of the ethics of informed consent, patients know they may be receiving a placebo, but many patients in a placebo group *believe* they are getting the real treatment when they're not, which creates expectancy. In other words, the expectation that you will feel differently leads you to feel differently.[17]

But expectation may not be the only factor contributing to the body's response. The second explanation for why people may get better is classical conditioning. We all know Pavlov's classic dog experiment. Not only did Pavlov's dog salivate in response to his Scooby Snack, he also started salivating when he heard the bell that accompanied it. The placebo effect may work in much the same way. If you're used to getting a real drug from a person in a white coat and subsequently getting better, then you may be conditioned to feel better by simply receiving a sugar pill from someone in a white coat.[18] This combination of expectation and conditioning creates measurable changes in brain activity and neurochemistry. Scientists have shown that placebo effects rely on complex neurobiological mechanisms involving neurotransmitters (endorphins, cannabinoids, and dopamine), as well as the activation of relevant areas of the brain (prefrontal cortex, anterior insula, rostral anterior cingulate cortex, and amygdala).[19] This suggests that anything we can do to mimic these neurobiological changes might alter perception of symptomatology.

The third explanation is that patients participating in clinical trials go through the ritual of treatment, and this ritual may have therapeutic benefits. Ted Kaptchuk, director of Harvard's Program in Placebo Studies and the Therapeutic Encounter (PiPS), says, "When you look at these studies that compare drugs with placebos, there is the entire environmental and ritual factor at work. You have to go to a clinic at certain times and be examined by medical professionals in white coats. You receive all kinds of exotic pills and undergo strange procedures. All this can have a profound impact on how the body perceives symptoms because you feel you are getting attention and care." Kaptchuk often makes the argument that the nurturing care of a respected authority figure may account as much for the placebo effect as positive belief, or even more. A patient in a clinical trial receives attention, support, and sometimes even healing touch, often delivered by an authority figure in a white coat, which has historically come to represent health and healing. We all want to feel seen, heard, even loved, and this alone may relieve symptoms and stimulate positive physiological change, again because of a mind-body-spirit link.

The fourth explanation for why people respond to placebos is that, while most studies try to screen out patients who are self-prescribing other treatments, a percentage of patients in clinical trials may still be surreptitiously seeking other treatments that may confound the data. If someone gets better while in a clinical trial, it's possible that the other treatments he or she has been sneaking under the table may be responsible for the improvement. This is true whether the patient is receiving the real treatment or the placebo. In either case, other treatments may be responsible for symptom relief that is then falsely attributed to either the drug or the placebo. After all, sick people are often experimenting with diet changes, supplements, and alternative medicine treatments, which are hard to screen out in clinical studies. How are we sure they're not getting better because of these other interventions?

The fifth explanation is that some patients may get better because the disease resolves itself on its own. After all, the body is a self-healing organism, constantly striving to return to homeostasis. So even if you stuck patients in a dark room, with no treatment or personal attention, a certain percentage of them might improve. Though there is controversy around this subject, a few scientists believe that the phenomenon of spontaneous remission is the only explanation for the placebo effect. Dr. Asbjørn Hróbjartsson and Dr. Peter Gøtzsche's *New England Journal of Medicine* article "Is the Placebo Powerless?" claims that we can't demonstrate a clear placebo effect unless studies also include a no-treatment group that gets neither the drug nor the sugar pill (which most don't).[20] In their study, they found little evidence of any meaningful placebo effect when no-treatment groups were studied, suggesting that it's not positive belief or nurturing care responsible for disease remission, but rather the natural history of the disease.[21] Others criticize this study, however, for its design flaws, claiming that comparing placebo groups from vastly different types of studies, evaluating completely different illnesses, is comparing apples and oranges, making interpretation of the combined data potentially misleading.[22]

While controversy exists among researchers, the general consensus is that the placebo effect is very real. It has even been reported in very young children and animals, suggesting that belief may be less important than we once thought. In the *New England Journal of Medicine*, Kaptchuk sums it up: "Placebo effects are improvements in patients' symptoms that are attributable to their participation in the therapeutic encounter, with its rituals, symbols, and interactions. These effects are distinct from those of discrete therapies and are precipitated by the contextual or environmental cues that surround medical interventions, both those that are fake and lacking in inherent therapeutic power and those with demonstrated efficacy. This diverse collection of signs and behaviors includes identifiable health-care paraphernalia and settings, emotional and cognitive engagement with clinicians, empathic and intimate witnessing, and the laying on of hands."[23]

What can we make of all this? Must we swallow fake pills or inject fake solutions in order to take advantage of the effects of expectation, conditioning, and ritual on symptom relief? Kaptchuk says that practicing self-help methods is one way. "Engaging in the ritual of healthy living—eating right, exercising, yoga, quality social time, meditating—probably provides some of the key ingredients of a placebo effect."[24]

The Physiology of the Placebo Effect

We know that the placebo effect is a real phenomenon. But what are the physiological mechanisms that explain how thoughts, feelings, and beliefs may translate into symptom relief? Researchers argue over the answer to this question, but several theories have been postulated. Thinking positively about getting well may stimulate natural endorphins, which help ameliorate symptoms, relieve pain, and lift your mood. The reverse is also true: when patients who responded positively to placebo were given the opioid blocker naloxone, which blocks natural endorphins, the placebo suddenly stopped being effective.[25]

Expecting you'll get better, being nurtured by caring clinical researchers, and engaging in the ritual of a therapeutic encounter may also relieve physiological stress, known to predispose the body to illness, and initiate physiological relaxation, which is necessary for the body's self-repair mechanisms to operate properly. As first described by Harvard professor Dr. Walter Cannon, the body is equipped with what Cannon named the stress response, also known as the fight-or-flight response, a survival mechanism that gets flipped on when your brain perceives a threat. When this hormonal cascade is triggered by a thought or emotion in the mind, such as fear, the hypothalamic-pituitary-adrenal (HPA) axis activates, thereby stimulating the sympathetic nervous system to race into overdrive, pumping up the body's cortisol and adrenaline levels. Over time, filling the body with these stress hormones can manifest as physical symptoms, predisposing the body to disease over time.

But as we'll discuss in more detail in Chapter 8, just as the stress response exists as a survival mechanism designed to help us stay alive in emergency situations, the body also has a counterbalancing relaxation response. When the relaxation response is elicited, stress hormones drop, health-inducing relaxation hormones that counter the stress hormones are released, the parasympathetic nervous system takes over, and the body returns to homeostasis. Even the most conventional medical doctors acknowledge that the body is fully equipped with an innate wisdom tuned in to an organizing intelligence that knows how to repair what breaks down in the body on a daily basis. Every day, we make and kill off cancer cells in our bodies. We fight off infectious agents and repair damaged cells and replace old tissues with fresh ones. But this inborn body wisdom only seems to operate at full capacity when the nervous system is in the parasympathetic "rest and repair" state. Anything that reduces stress and elicits a relaxation response not only alleviates the symptoms the stress response can cause but also frees the body to do what it does naturally—heal itself.

Positive belief, nurturing care, and the ritual of the therapeutic encounter may also alter the immune system. People treated with placebos may experience boosts in immune function resulting from flipping off the stress response and initiating the relaxation response. Placebos may also suppress the immune system when appropriate. In one study, rats were given the immunosuppressive drug cyclophosphamide (mixed with saccharin water). Then the drug itself was removed, and the rats were fed only the saccharin water (a placebo). Lo and behold: their immune systems stayed objectively suppressed, even when they were no longer getting the drug, suggesting that even rats may respond to the placebo effect with measurable physiological immune responses.[26] This paradoxical reaction of the immune system to placebo influences suggests that the innate body wisdom may even know best when to mount an immune response, as when an infection is brewing, and when to suppress an immune response, as in the case of autoimmune diseases.

The placebo effect may also decrease the body's acute phase response, a type of inflammatory response that leads to pain, swelling, fever, lethargy, apathy, and loss of appetite.[27]

The mind-body-spirit link may also be mediated by executive functions of the prefrontal cortex of the brain. The fact that placebo responses are disrupted in people with Alzheimer's disease supports this theory.[28] Many with Alzheimer's disease fail to respond to placebos, supporting the idea that an area of the brain related to expectancy, which may be damaged in a neurological disease state, affects whether a patient responds to placebos. Evolutionary biologist Robert Trivers says that what the brain expects to happen in the near future affects its physiological state. Trivers suggests that those with Alzheimer's don't experience a placebo effect because they are unable to anticipate the future, so their minds cannot physiologically prepare for it.

Placebo responsiveness also correlates to activation of dopamine in the nucleus accumbens, a region of the brain involved in reward mechanisms. Scientists studied the brains of people after they were given money to see how much dopamine they released in the nucleus accumbens. The more the nucleus accumbens responded to a monetary reward, the more likely those patients were to get well with a placebo.[29]

Whatever the mechanism, it's clear that the mind and body communicate through hormones and neurotransmitters that originate in the brain and then leave the brain to signal other parts of the body. So it should come as no surprise to us that what we think and how we feel can translate into physiological changes in the rest of the body.

But it kinda does, doesn't it? At least in my medical school, there wasn't much talk about how our thoughts, feelings, and expectations affect the health of the body. Yet, if they do, why are we not more careful about what we put into our minds? But I'm getting ahead of myself. We'll talk more about how to keep your mind, body, and spirit healthy in Part Two of this book.

Are All Diseases Equally Placebo Responsive?

The next question that arose in my quest to understand the placebo effect was whether placebos work for every disease. Do all symptoms and diseases respond to placebos, or are there only certain types of diseases that respond?

What I found is that nearly every clinical trial demonstrates a placebo effect, but some health conditions appear to be more placebo responsive than others. Placebos seem to be most effective when given to patients with immune system conditions such as allergies, endocrine disorders such as diabetes, inflammatory conditions such as colitis, mental health conditions such as anxiety and depression, nervous system disorders such as Parkinson's and insomnia, cardiac symptoms such as angina, respiratory conditions such as asthma and cough, and, especially, pain disorders.

But do placebos work to treat cancer? Heart attacks? Strokes? Liver failure? Kidney disease?

In my research, I couldn't find much data to answer this question, perhaps because treating conditions like these in a clinical trial with a placebo would be considered unethical. With these kinds of life-threatening conditions, new treatments are usually studied against gold-standard treatments that already exist and have been proven to have at least some efficacy. So it's hard to know the limits of what will and won't respond to a placebo.

The American Cancer Society takes a clear stand: "In studies where doctors are looking at whether a tumor shrinks, placebos have very little, if any, effect. . . . The bottom line is that placebos don't cure."[30] In a review article published in the *New England Journal of Medicine*, placebo researcher Kaptchuk concluded, "Though placebos may provide relief, they rarely cure."[31] While physiological changes have been observed in response to placebo treatment, placebos seem to resolve symptoms more than they resolve the disease itself. This is not to suggest that spontaneous remissions do not happen. We know they do. We just don't fully understand the mechanism by which such seeming miracles happen.

While the placebo effect remains mysterious, what we do know is that placebos seem to work best by altering the patient's *perception* of physical symptoms, which paves the way for changing our relationship to what we perceive as suffering. Since so many chronically ill people are plagued with symptoms that interfere with quality of life, I became curious about what sick people could do to alter their perception of the symptoms that cause suffering. Are there ways we can be proactive about helping the nervous system relax so the hormonal milieu of natural healing can be optimized? If we shift both our perception of suffering and the physiology of how our cells and organs are bathed with the hormones of stress or healing, what might be possible then?

Unlocking the Mystery of Spontaneous Remission

While I doubted that I would every fully unravel the medical mystery of what seem like miraculous cures, I was dogged in my search for clues. I found my next lead at a holiday cocktail party at the Institute of Noetic Sciences (IONS) in Petaluma, California, where I was sipping a glass of wine and chatting about my research with Marilyn Schlitz, Ph.D., who was the president of IONS at the time. When I told her my conundrum, Marilyn smiled at me with a look that said, "No problem!" and referred me to an online database that Caryle Hirshberg and Brendan O'Regan had compiled called the Spontaneous Remission Project. This database includes an impressive annotated bibliography of 3,500 references from more than 800 journals in 20 different languages, documenting cases of unexplainable spontaneous disease remission. They defined spontaneous remission as "the disappearance, complete or incomplete, of a disease or cancer without medical treatment or treatment that is considered inadequate to produce the resulting disappearance of disease symptoms or tumor."[32]

The bibliography includes some astonishing cases. An HIV-positive patient became HIV-negative. One woman with untreated metastatic breast cancer had breast, lung, and femur tumors that resolved spontaneously. The plaques blocking a man's coronary arteries disappeared without treatment. A man's brain aneurysm disappeared. A man with a gunshot wound in the brain recovered with no treatment. A woman with cardiomyopathy in heart failure got better. A woman with thyroid disease experienced a spontaneous cure.[33]

I also became aware of two similarly titled books written in the 1960s, Boyd's *The Spontaneous Regression of Cancer* and Everson and Cole's *Spontaneous Regression of Cancer*, which spawned an increase in the number of such case studies reported in the medical literature.

As I read through case study after case study of spontaneous disease remission, I felt my heart race with excitement. For the most part, the case studies didn't address *how* the spontaneous remissions happened. The patients weren't interviewed about whether they believed they would get well, whether they were taking placebos, or whether they had done anything else remarkable to heal themselves.

But they did give me proof that almost no disease can be called "incurable." Many of the health conditions from which patients spontaneously got well were the kinds of illnesses I was taught were terminal and untreatable. Clearly, I had been taught wrong.

I wasn't the only one whose curiosity was sparked by case studies like this, wondering why conventional medicine wasn't asking more questions about those outliers who experienced cures from seemingly "incurable" diseases. At the same time as I was hounding the halls of IONS, Kelly Turner was getting her Ph.D. at the University of California, Berkeley, after traveling the world to interview people who experienced "radical remissions" from stage 4 cancers that had been either untreated by conventional medicine or given treatment deemed to be inadequate for cure. Her book *Radical Remission*, compiling her stories and conclusions about the nine factors these patients had in common, was released shortly after the first edition of *Mind Over Medicine* was published. (Review Dr. Turner's nine factors, including one new one, in Appendix B.)

Years later, I would also meet physician, ordained minister, and Harvard instructor Jeffrey Rediger, M.D., M.Div., who, in addition to practicing medicine, received a master's in divinity from the Princeton Theological Seminary, giving him the perfect credentials to research the intersection of science and spirituality. He published a book, *Cured: The Life-Changing Science of Spontaneous Healing*, detailing the findings of his research into the health outliers who have experienced unusual health outcomes. I was relieved and grateful to meet another legitimate academician with a tendency to nerd out like I did about the mind-body-spirit connection. I discovered that, since 2003, he has been collecting stories of radical remission, as Kelly Turner and I had. With degrees in both medicine and theology, he stood with one foot in two worlds, bridging the scientific explanation of such phenomena as "spontaneous remissions" or "placebo effects" on the one side of the bridge and holding the tension with the religious world on the other side that would classify such things as "miracles" or "spiritual healing." As he writes, "These terms are all black boxes that have not been unpacked by the tools of modern science."[34] He has been tracking these cases for so long that he's had the opportunity to see how some of these health outliers fare over the long haul–stories of better-than-expected outcomes in patients with pancreatic cancer, the worst forms of brain cancer, idiopathic pulmonary fibrosis, and other potentially fatal diseases.

Our shared interest would lead to hours of brain dumping and a new friendship. Dr. Rediger expressed frustration about why we obsess over outliers in other disciplines. We rigorously study the Steve Jobs of the business world or the Serena Williams of the tennis world, trying to understand what makes them such high achievers.

But why don't we study the high achievers in the arena of health with equal rigor and curiosity? What is it about radical remissions that makes most doctors and scientists so uncomfortable that we lose our scientific objectivity? Is it just that we're so uncomfortable admitting that we simply don't understand the mechanisms by which radical remissions happen?

Kelly Turner, Jeffrey Rediger, and I all marveled at how the conventional medical community responded to health outliers. One patient said to me, "He wasn't even curious about what I'd done. In fact, he seemed mad at me for proving him wrong when he told me I had six months to live." Another wrote me a letter about her doctor's response. She said, "She insisted it must have been a misdiagnosis, since this disease cannot be cured. I was standing there in front of her with the medical evidence that my disease was gone, and she literally could not even look me in the eye. I think it was just too confronting to her. If I was cured, her whole worldview might have to change. I think she just couldn't handle being wrong. If she was wrong about this, what else was she wrong about? I wonder if someone shamed her when she got something wrong when she was a little girl. That's what it felt like, like she was a scared little girl who got a bad grade on a test and got punished for getting the answers wrong. I almost felt sorry for her, but mostly, I felt angry that she couldn't even give me a high five or validate that my efforts had been rewarded with a miracle."

I felt a lot of intense emotions in myself when patients told me their stories. I found myself apologizing on behalf of doctors I didn't even know, feeling everything from rage to grief to guilt to relief to compassion to gratitude. By this point in my journey, I was getting used to feeling a lot of mixed feelings. Parts of me were excited and passionately devoted to this mission, feeling a strong sense of fulfillment and a devotion to my calling. Other parts were resisting the journey. I started experiencing somatic symptoms, as if I had a perpetual case of belly butterflies. I felt inexplicably frightened, as if I might get burned at the stake or at least rejected by my peers in the medical community that had once embraced and celebrated my achievements and contributions. I felt a lot of sadness and shame when I thought about all the patients I might have harmed with my own ignorance.

At one point I had to go out under the vast, starry sky of a moonless night and just gaze at the enormity of an unknowable universe while hugging myself and rocking. Somehow, this calmed my nervous system and helped me carry on. In spite of my resistance, I knew I was not going to stop diving down the rabbit hole. I had passed the point of no return. I started seeing a therapist to help me heal the parts of me that were resisting, and I found that when I loved and accepted my resistant parts, they relaxed and let me continue on my journey so I could help guide you on yours.

I had proven to myself, without a shadow of a doubt, that the mind-body-spirit connection *can* heal the body, at least some of the time. I even had some semblance of a logical physiological explanation for how it happens. But I knew I was only just beginning to understand the complexities of these mysteries, and I still didn't understand how to harness this power in order to help people prevent illness and treat disease. So I dug deeper.

CHAPTER 2

THE SUREFIRE WAY TO MAKE YOURSELF SICK AND PREVENT DISEASE REMISSION

Never affirm or repeat about your health what you do not wish to be true.

— RALPH WALDO TRINE

After learning so much about the benefits of the placebo effect, I became curious about whether the opposite was also true. If positive expectations, the nurturing care of a clinician, and the ritual of the therapeutic encounter can heal the body, does that mean negative beliefs and harsh care from an insensitive clinician can harm the body?

I first wanted to examine the role of negative expectations on the body's physiology. Do people have the power to think themselves sick?

Turns out they do. Researchers in San Diego examined the death records of almost 30,000 Chinese Americans and compared them to over 400,000 randomly selected white people. What they found was that Chinese Americans, but not whites, die significantly earlier than normal (by as much as five years) if they have a combination of disease and birth year that Chinese astrology and Chinese medicine consider ill-fated. The researchers found that the more strongly the

Chinese Americans attached to traditional Chinese traditions, the earlier they died. When they examined the data, they concluded that the reduction in life expectancy could not be explained by genetic factors, the lifestyle choices or behavior of the patient, the skill of the doctor, or any other variable.

Why did the Chinese Americans die younger? The researchers concluded that they died younger not because they had Chinese genes but because they had Chinese expectations. They believed they would die younger because the stars had hexed them. And their negative belief manifested as a shorter life.[1]

More studies suggest that negative beliefs affect your health. One study showed that 79 percent of medical students report developing symptoms suggestive of the illnesses they are studying.[2] Because they get paranoid and think they'll get sick, they do.

I know this from personal experience. I was a first-year medical student, studying the numerous ways the body can run amuck, burning the midnight oil to memorize the litany of pathological processes that can lead to thousands of different illnesses—everything from porphyria to dengue fever to osteogenesis imperfecta to narcolepsy.

Then suddenly I felt something crawling under my skin. I figured it must have been a guinea worm, creeping into my subcutaneous space, ready to break through the skin at any moment and poke its little head out. I also noticed that my feet felt numb when I first woke up in the morning. I was 100 percent certain it was leprosy. The palms of my hands had a speckled pattern that couldn't be anything but fifth disease. And the night sweats, which left me with soaking wet pajamas, could only mean one thing: malaria.

I didn't wind up with leprosy or guinea worms, but as I described in the introduction, I did wind up with multiple chronic health conditions that were diagnosed during my medical education, and I strongly suspect my negative beliefs about my health had something to do with it.

I wasn't the only medical student who was afflicted with a whole host of physical symptoms. In fact, the student health clinic didn't seem the least bit surprised to see me and my fellow students, traipsing through just before finals with bizarre complaints and a slew of self-diagnoses. Not only had the doctors and nurses staffing these clinics heard similar complaints from years of experience caring for medical students, they also informed me that the syndrome had actually been given a name: "medstudentitis," or, more formally, "medical student disease."

Think Sick, Be Sick

Whether you're a Chinese American, a medical student, or *you*, focusing your attention on illness has been scientifically proven to make you sick. Excessive knowledge about what can go wrong with the body can actually harm you. The more you focus on the infinite ways in which the body can break down, the more likely you are to experience physical symptoms.

Scientists call this phenomenon the nocebo effect. While the placebo effect demonstrates the power of positive thinking, expectation, hope, and nurturing care, the nocebo effect demonstrates the power of negative belief. While a placebo was traditionally prescribed to help the patient feel better, the term *nocebo* (Latin for "I shall harm") was introduced to differentiate the pleasing effects of placebos from the harmful effects inert treatments can induce.

For example, if you tell patients in a clinical trial they will be given a pill that will relieve their pain, there's a good chance the pain will go away, even if they're given only a sugar pill. But if you warn them that the treatment might cause nausea and vomiting, there's a high likelihood they'll puke, even when they never got the real drug. In fact, many patients who don't understand the nocebo effect assume they're getting the real drug when they start experiencing the side effects they have been warned they might experience should they be randomized to the treatment group. Little do they know that the nocebo effect is as real as the placebo effect. In other words, the presence of side effects doesn't indicate that they are getting the real treatment any more than the resolution of symptoms proves they're getting the real deal.

In *Love, Medicine & Miracles*, Dr. Bernie Siegel cites one study showing that patients in a control group for a new chemotherapy drug were given nothing but saline, yet they were warned it could be chemotherapy, and 30 percent of them lost their hair.[3] In another study, hospitalized patients were given sugar water and told it would make them throw up. Eighty percent of them vomited.[4]

In a study published in *The Pavlovian Journal of Biological Science*, 34 college students were hooked up to monitors and told that an electric current would be passed through their heads. Study participants were warned that they might experience a headache as a side effect. Although not one volt of current was actually used, more than two-thirds of the students reported headaches.[5]

Even thoughts about death seem to play out. According to Dr. Herbert Benson, a Harvard professor and the president of Mind/Body Medical Institute in Boston, "Surgeons are wary of people who are convinced that they will die. There are examples of studies done on people undergoing surgery who almost want to die to re-contact a loved one. Close to 100 percent of people under those circumstances die."[6]

Patients about to undergo surgery who were "convinced" of their impending death were compared to another group of patients who were merely "unusually apprehensive" about death. While the apprehensive bunch fared pretty well, those who were convinced they were going to die usually did. Similarly, women who believed they were prone to heart disease were four times more likely to die of heart disease than those who did not believe they would. It's not because these women had poorer diets, higher blood pressure, higher cholesterol, or stronger family histories than the women who didn't get heart disease. The only difference between the two groups was their beliefs.[7]

One fascinating case study described a psychiatric patient with a split personality. As one personality, the patient was not diabetic, and her blood glucose levels were normal. However, the moment she became her alter ego, she *believed* she was diabetic, and she literally *became* diabetic. Her entire physiology shifted. Her blood sugars rose, and from all medical evidence, she was, in fact, diabetic. When her personality flipped back, her blood sugars returned to normal.[8]

Psychiatrist Bennett Braun, author of *The Treatment of Multiple Personality Disorder*, describes several similar cases. Timmy, for example, drinks orange juice uneventfully. But Timmy is only one of one patient's many personalities, and while Timmy can drink orange juice without consequence, all the other personalities are allergic to orange juice and break out into blistering hives at the slightest sip. If, however, Timmy comes back in the midst of an allergic reaction, the hives instantly resolve, and the water-filled blisters begin to subside.[9]

Nocebos can result in sickness, and even death, when the patient expects such an outcome. Scientific studies investigating the nocebo effect can be ethically challenging, since it's hard to get institutional review boards to approve studies designed to intentionally make patients feel worse. Because of this, there is less data to support the existence of the nocebo effect than there is for the placebo effect. Most of what we know about the nocebo effect comes as a side effect of clinical trials that include placebos.

When patients in double-blinded clinical trials are warned about the side effects they may experience if they're given the real drug, approximately 25 percent do experience side effects, sometimes severe, even when they're only taking sugar pills.[10] Those treated with nothing more than placebos often report fatigue, vomiting, muscle weakness, colds, ringing in the ears, taste disturbances, memory disturbances, and other symptoms that shouldn't result from a sugar pill.

Interestingly, these nocebo complaints aren't random; they tend to arise in response to the side-effect warnings on the actual drug or treatment. The mere suggestion that a patient may experience negative symptoms in response to a medication (or a sugar pill) may be a self-fulfilling prophecy. For example, if you tell a patient treated with a placebo he might experience nausea, he's likely to feel nauseous. If you suggest that he might get a headache, he may. In other words, the power of suggestion is *powerful*.[11]

The nocebo effect is probably most obvious in "voodoo death," when a person is cursed and told he or she will die, then dies.[12] The notion of voodoo death doesn't just apply to witch doctors in tribal cultures. The literature shows that patients believed to be terminal who are mistakenly informed that they have only a few months to live have died within their given time frame, even when autopsy findings reveal no physiological explanation for the early death.[13]

Dr. Sanford Cohen described an AIDS patient who experts believe died because he overheard his mother saying she wanted him to die. The patient, whose mother learned on the same day that her son was both gay and afflicted with AIDS, openly prayed outside his ICU room that he would die because of the shame he brought on her. One hour later, he did die, much to the doctor's surprise, since the patient had not appeared to be terminal.[14]

Some believe that those who suffer from premenstrual syndrome (PMS) symptoms may be victims of a sort of nocebo effect. Because they believe they will experience symptoms before their menses, they do. One study of women debilitated by PMS engineered a scheme to trick the study subjects into thinking their periods would come at a different time than they normally expected by giving them an inert pill they were told would alter the timing of their menses. For example, a woman who normally gets her period mid-month and suffers from PMS for three days before her menses was told she would menstruate on the first of the month instead.

What happened? Even though the timing of her period didn't actually change, she got her PMS early that month because she *believed* she would.[15]

Nocebo symptoms can manifest in large groups as well as individuals. For example, after the nuclear power plant disaster in Japan following the 2011 tsunami, people with no evidence of radiation exposure reported symptoms of radiation poisoning as far away as the United States. Similarly, thousands of people with no evidence of disease reported symptoms of swine flu after the media blasted reports of the epidemic all over television, newspapers, and the Internet. Similar "epidemics" have been reported in workplaces, schools, and towns where gas leaks, strange odors, or insect bites have been reported in the media.[16]

So how does this happen? How can someone shed hair when given saline? How can they vomit when given sugar water? How can they become diabetic or allergic to orange juice just by switching personalities? What is occurring, both in the brain and in the body? I kept digging to find my answers.

Scientists believe the nocebo effect is caused primarily by activation of the same stress response the placebo effect relieves. When a patient is cursed, either by a witch doctor, a family member, or a modern physician, the stress of the bad news stimulates the stress response. For example, when patients were told they would experience pain (but were given only an inert substance), the HPA axis was stimulated, increasing cortisol levels. Both pain and excess stimulation of the HPA axis were experienced and then relieved with Valium, indicating that a stress mechanism was at play.[17]

Some also theorize that those who are pronounced ill may become so despondent that they simply stop caring for themselves and suffer the consequences of poor self-care. They may also become depressed, and as I'll discuss in Chapter 7, the link between depression and poor health is very clear.

Further support for the idea that our beliefs may translate into physiological changes in our bodies comes from the laboratories of those studying the field of molecular biology called epigenetics, meaning "above the genes." So what's "above the genes" when we talk about epigenetic control?

Yup. You guessed it. The mind, or you might even say "consciousness." As it turns out, while you can't change your DNA, you may be able to utilize the power of your consciousness to alter how your DNA expresses itself. Traditional genetic determinism, as elucidated by Watson and Crick, who discovered the DNA double helix, supports the notion that everything in the body is controlled by our genes—that, essentially, our genes are our destiny. If this is true, we are literally victims of our genes. Heart disease, breast cancer, diabetes, alcoholism, depression, high cholesterol—you name it. If it runs in your family, you're basically hosed.

The dogma of genetic determinism, as it has been traditionally taught, is simple: you're born with your DNA, which then gets replicated as RNA before being translated into proteins that determine every minute detail of your body's appearance, function, and tendencies toward either health or disease. But the study of epigenetics brings the whole notion of genetic determinism into question. This doesn't mean we are blank slates. Our genes do tend to influence our health, but we are not at the mercy of our genes in the way the traditional genetic determinists used to believe. The truth lies somewhere between being victims of our genes and being unaffected by them. What is now clear in the evolving field of epigenetics is that your thoughts, expectations, and feelings affect how your genes express themselves by impacting the internal environment of the body, as do other external environmental factors, such as what you eat or what you're exposed to in your living environment.

Sadly, most of us are not programmed to have positive thoughts, expectations, and feelings about our health. Instead, from the time we are children, our minds are programmed with beliefs that sabotage our efforts to become optimally healthy and happy. Beliefs like "I catch colds easily," "I always overeat," "I probably won't live very long," and "Cancer runs in my family" cause the mind to trigger physiological stress responses that impact how the genes express themselves. These programmed beliefs that arise from childhood apply not just to physical health. They also apply to deeper and broader self-limiting beliefs ("I'm not worthy," "I'm not smart enough," "I don't deserve to make a lot of money," "I'm a loser," "Nobody will ever love me"). Negative core beliefs about health can also go beyond inherited beliefs, arising from traumas in this lifetime and impacting how our genes express themselves.

Negative Core Beliefs about Health

Advanced Integrative Therapy (AIT) founder Asha Clinton, Ph.D., developed a list of negative core beliefs that commonly underlie health challenges. Negative core beliefs result from traumas earlier in life and can be difficult to clear without treating the underlying traumas, which is why affirmations alone rarely work to permanently change limiting beliefs. Some examples of negative core beliefs that can impede healing include the following:

- My body betrayed me.
- I'd rather be sick than feel my emotions.
- I want to opt out of the aspects of life I can't cope with.
- I caused my disease.
- If God loved me, I wouldn't have my disease.

- My body is spoiled and broken.
- I cannot get well.
- I need to be sick so [fill in the blank] will take care of me.
- I need to be sick so I don't have to [name the thing to be avoided].

*Learn more about the AIT approach to negative core beliefs at http://ait.institute.

A Closer Look at Epigenetics

Negative core beliefs about health and other aspects of life are typically the result of the everyday traumas we all experience, so healing the traumas that lead to such beliefs becomes an essential part of any treatment plan for someone suffering from life-threatening or chronic disease. Because they create so much interference in the nervous system and the body's energetic system, core beliefs like these can actually change how your brain communicates with the rest of your body, thereby altering the body's biochemistry. It's not just your brain that is subject to this kind of plasticity. While you can't change your DNA, cell biologist and author of *The Biology of Belief* Dr. Bruce Lipton asserts that you may be able to change how your DNA is expressed based on what you believe.[18]

Your genetic code is like a blueprint that can be interpreted in millions of different ways. Before the Human Genome Project, biologists assumed that we had at least 120,000 genes, one gene for every protein made in the body. So researchers were baffled when they discovered that we only have approximately 25,000 genes, which can express themselves in a variety of different ways.

In fact, we now know that each of those 25,000 genes can express itself in at least 30,000 ways via regulatory proteins that are influenced by environmental signals. Studies have even shown that environmental factors can override certain genetic mutations, effectively changing how the DNA is expressed. These altered genes can then be passed down to offspring, allowing the offspring to express healthier characteristics, even though they still carry the genetic mutation.[19]

The study of epigenetic control is revolutionizing how we think about genes. We used to think that some people were blessed with "good genes," while others were cursed with what some in the medical community insensitively refer to as "piss-poor protoplasm." In fact, few diseases result from a single gene mutation. Less than 2 percent of diseases, such as cystic fibrosis, Huntington's chorea, and beta-thalassemia, result from a single faulty gene, and only about 5 percent of cancer and cardiac disease patients can attribute their diseases to heredity.[20] Scientists are now learning that the genome is far more responsive to the environment of the cell than genetic determinism suggests. This means that the majority of disease processes can be explained by environmental factors to which the cells are exposed, things such as nutrition, hormonal changes, the biochemistry of peace in our nervous systems, and even the hormones of love. We need not be victims of our DNA.

The Body as a Petri Dish

Intrigued by what I had learned in Lipton's book but curious to know more, I interviewed him. He explained to me that in his bench research as a cell biologist, he worked with pluripotential stem cells, cells that can become anything when they grow up. He placed one cell in a Petri dish, where it was nourished with cell culture medium as it divided into many genetically identical cells. Lipton then split the cells into three Petri dishes and exposed them to three different culture media (the environment). What he discovered was that the environment to which the cell was exposed determined whether the cell became a muscle cell or a fat cell or a bone cell. Even though all the cells were genetically identical, they expressed themselves differently. The final outcome of the genetically identical DNA was its expression as radically different cells.

What controlled the fate of the cells? Not the genetics. They were all genetically identical. The sole difference was the environment to which the same DNA was exposed. The cellular environment also determined whether or not the cells stayed healthy. Cells exposed to a "good" environment (a healthy cell medium) enjoyed optimal health, while those exposed to a "bad" environment (an unhealthy cell medium) got sick.

Lipton said, "If I were an allopathic physician of cells, I'd diagnose the cells in the bad medium as sick. Surely, they need medicine. But that's not really what they need. If you take the sick cells out of the bad environment and put them back into the good environment, they naturally recover—without medicine."

One day, as he was observing the cells in his lab, Lipton had an epiphany. He realized that the human body is no different from the cells in his lab. Lipton said, "The human is nothing more than a skin-covered Petri dish with a community of 50 trillion cells. Whether the cells are in our bodies or in the Petri dish doesn't matter. The culture medium of the cells in our bodies is the blood that bathes and feeds them. If we change the composition of the blood, it's the same as changing the culture medium of the cells. So what controls the composition of the blood? The brain is the chemist changing the environment to which our cells are exposed. The brain releases neuropeptides, hormones, growth factors, and other chemicals, akin to adding chemicals to a Petri dish with a pipette, thereby changing the cell medium."

When I asked him how belief can change the cellular environment, Lipton explained that the brain is perception, but the mind is interpretation. It's all about how the mind interprets a life event. For example, you can open your eyes and see a person. (This is your brain's objective perception.) Your mind may then recognize this person as someone you love. (This is the mind's interpretation.) The brain then releases oxytocin, dopamine, endorphins, and other positive chemicals that provide the healthy cell medium of the whole body's cells via the blood.

If, on the other hand, you open your eyes and see a person (the perception), and your mind interprets this person as scary, the brain releases stress hormones and other fear chemicals that damage the cells. Lipton says, "When we shift the mind's interpretation of illness from fear and danger to positive belief, the brain responds biochemically, the blood changes the body's cell culture, and the cells change on a biological level."

I had my own aha moment when Dr. Lipton explained this to me. Suddenly, it was all making sense. It all kept coming back to the hormones and neurotransmitters the brain spits out depending on whether the mind interprets something as positive (as it does with the placebo effect) or negative (as with the nocebo effect). When our beliefs are hopeful and optimistic, the mind releases chemicals that put the body in a state of physiological rest, controlled primarily by the parasympathetic nervous system, and in this state of rest, the body's natural self-repair mechanisms are free to get to work fixing what's broken in the body.

If, however, the mind is looping the kind of negative core beliefs that plague so many of us, the brain perceives these as a threat. Whether these painful beliefs relate to your health, your love life, your relationships with your family of origin, your worth, your financial security, your ability to express your talent and fulfill your calling, or your sense of disconnection from a spiritual Source, as far as the brain is concerned, there's a lion running after you, so it's time to fight, flee, or freeze. When the body's stress responses are activated, the body isn't concerned with long-term issues like cellular rejuvenation, self-repair, fending off infections, or fighting the effects of aging. It's too busy preparing you to run away from the lion. No point putting your immune cells to work chewing up stray cancer cells or turning over fresh new cells in the body if you're about to get eaten.

Over time, these negative beliefs that repetitively trigger the stress response take their toll. The cellular environment gets poisoned with stress hormones. It's no wonder the body gets sick and has a hard time repairing itself.

What Happened in the Womb Matters

Environmental and emotional factors can affect how DNA expresses itself as far back as when we are in the womb. A wide range of diseases that affect adults—like osteoporosis and depression—have been linked to prenatal and perinatal developmental influences.[21] Once again, this throws the whole notion of genetic determinism, a limited view of genetics Lipton calls *gene myopia*, into question.

In *Life in the Womb*, Dr. Peter Nathanielsz explains that there is mounting evidence that programming of lifetime health by the conditions of the womb is as important as, if not more important than, our genes in determining how we perform mentally and physically during life.[22]

The affection we receive in infancy also shapes our baby brains, changing receptors in the brain, which affect the thermostat of how the adult body responds to stressful stimuli, which in turn can translate into disease in later life. In fact, lack of mother-baby bonding in early life doesn't affect only our bodies; it may threaten our whole society, predisposing it to depression, aggression, and drug abuse, thereby affecting the peace of an entire culture.[23]

In other words, our parents can shape our health when we're barely more than a twinkle in their eyes. A whole host of chronic diseases can develop as the result of adverse environmental and emotional influences we experience as fetuses.[24]

Your Subconscious Mind and Positive Thinking

Our parents also shape the beliefs that reside in our subconscious minds. Negative core beliefs we observe in our parents get involuntarily programmed into our subconscious minds at a young age, beliefs like "You're weak" or "You're going to wind up fat and saddled with diabetes when you grow up." Your subconscious mind gets filled with beliefs you download from parents, teachers, and others who influence you early in life, filling your mind with the programs that will run your life unless you get help reprogramming your subconscious mind. Usually, by the age of six, these programs have been written, and few people ever make efforts to examine and rewrite their subconscious programming. Given that we have no control over how this powerful part of our brain gets programmed by situational and developmental traumas when we're children, it's no wonder most people struggle to change limiting and self-sabotaging beliefs that can harm not just their health but all aspects of their lives.

Even if you're consciously vigilant about repeating all your positive, hopeful affirmations, you operate from the subconscious mind 95 percent of the time. These habitual negative beliefs, which kick in anytime we're not focusing our attention on positive thoughts, become the default. They operate when we're sleeping, when we're working, or anytime we're not consciously repeating our positive affirmations. Such beliefs may then activate a type of nocebo effect, since if the subconscious mind believes we will get sick, the brain perceives a threat, and the stress response is involuntarily and unconsciously triggered. Next thing you know, your body is busy running away from that perceived lion again, and the body suffers.

The power of the subconscious mind explains why positive thinking only gets you so far. How many times have you read self-help books, taken workshops, made New Year's resolutions, and vowed to improve your life, only to realize a year later that your life is no better? Since the conscious mind is only functioning 5 percent of the time, it has little power to overcome the weighty influence of the subconscious mind. To effect lasting changes in belief, you must change your beliefs not just at the level of the conscious mind but also in the subconscious mind. In order to change your beliefs permanently, you'll also need to treat the traumas that caused those beliefs to run on autopilot in your subconscious mind. Otherwise, you're just decorating a pile of poo with cream cheese icing.

Anytime we talk about positive or negative beliefs, we need to take care also not to valence beliefs or the emotions they activate into "good" or "bad." Notwithstanding all the good it's done, one destructive side effect of the positive psychology movement is that people tend to become frightened of the harmful effects of negative core beliefs or painful emotions, which only activates more stress responses! My mentor Rachel Naomi Remen, M.D., said, "I must confess that I find the notion of 'positive' emotions a disturbing concept and perhaps even a dangerous one. At best, it implies that there is a way to live, a certain set of attitudes, that may guarantee survival. At worst, the concept of positive emotions can degenerate into self-tyranny and may lead the individual into some kind of mind control. Many people now seem to fear harboring 'negative' emotions or 'wrong' thoughts in the same way people used to fear having evil thoughts."

Empathy researcher Karla McLaren would agree. In *The Art of Empathy*, she makes the case that every emotion is a necessary, useful call to action that brings with it gifts. Our invitation is to do our homework to become intimate with these emotions and become conscious of why they arrive and how they're here to help. For example, anger protects our boundaries, hopefully without violating the boundaries of others, and helps us lessen our attachments to people who treat us poorly. Fear is related to intuition, clarity, instinct, and attentiveness. It arises in the presence of change, uncertainty, and potential physical hazards, helping you focus on the present moment so you can sense danger and respond to what's happening appropriately. Sadness brings the gift of release, helping us let go of something that isn't working anyway, preparing us for grief when something has been lost irretrievably and needs to be mourned.

Such a spacious, nondemonizing relationship to all emotions is consistent with family therapist Richard Schwartz's Internal Family Systems (IFS) model. If you saw the fabulous Pixar movie *Inside Out*, you already have a sense of the IFS model. If you haven't seen it, the moral of the story after the little girl protagonist's parents move her away from her childhood home is (spoiler alert!) that sadness arrives for a reason and helps her get the love, attention, and comfort she needs so she can let go of what has been irretrievably lost. The Joy character within her tries to make her cast everything with a silver lining, but no amount of the "positive psychology" or "spiritual bypassing" Joy attempts helps the little girl move through her grief. Only letting sadness feel sad ultimately heals her and helps her move on.

How does that fit in with negative core beliefs? Well, such beliefs usually arise early in our lives as the result of unhealed traumas that are buried in our subconscious minds. In order to heal, release, and shift those beliefs, we have to do what we try so hard to avoid doing—become aware of the traumas that are running unbidden in our systems, expose ourselves to those painful feelings, and then utilize cutting-edge trauma treatments so we can clear those traumas from the subconscious mind and free ourselves to create the conditions of healing in the body, mind, and spirit. Once those traumas are treated, the negative core beliefs that arise as the result of such traumas have the potential to be shifted—quickly and permanently. Otherwise, if we only put a cheerful face over hurting parts, those painful emotions and negative core beliefs will keep running on autopilot underneath the surface of our awareness, interfering with our ability to achieve optimal health and happiness.

Be Mindful of How You Program Children

Many of us were programmed to have disempowering thoughts about our health at an early age. Few of our parents taught us that our minds have the power to heal and harm our own bodies. Instead, as my literary agent Michele Martin once said to me, "I thought my body was none of my business." Such beliefs leave us at the mercy of experts, powerless to influence our health outcomes if the doctor says, "There's nothing more I can do."

As children, most of us learn that when the body gets sick, we must go to the doctor and get treated. When a child falls and skins her knee, rarely does the parent say, "Okay, honey. Now your knee can focus on healing itself." No! We race off to get ointments and Band-Aids. There's nothing wrong with ointments and Band-Aids, but they feed into the child's erroneous belief that the body is dependent on treatments that come from the outside rather than the self-repair mechanisms our bodies all have naturally. The truth is that the ointments and Band-Aids keep the wound safe while the body does the heavy lifting of closing an open wound, just as a cast placed on a fractured bone or a bone surgery only stabilizes the bone so the bone can repair itself.

Imagine if parents programmed impressionable young subconscious minds to believe we have self-healing superpowers to fight disease and activate health, instead of teaching us that illness must be treated by dosing us up with medication or hauling us off to the doctor's office for a shot every time we get sick. Imagine how optimally healthy our subconscious minds could be if we were set up early in childhood to believe in the body's potential to facilitate all kinds of miracles.

What I've learned has changed how I parent my daughter, Siena. When she was three or four, before I learned what I now know, Siena's father, Matt, would joke with Siena when she got sick or injured. Mimicking an ambulance siren, he would race around the room with her in his arms, yelling, "Quick! Somebody call the ambulance! We have to take Siena to the kid factory so we can get her a new leg" (or lip or nose). She would laugh, and we would cover her injury with a Band-Aid or take her to the doctor. But the underlying message we were programming into her subconscious mind was "You have to go to the kid factory in order to get better." With that kind of programming, it would be hard for her adult self to accept that the body can heal itself.

Until I started researching the self-healing process, Matt and I had no idea we might be inadvertently affecting Siena's health and well-being. Equally certain, my own mother never wanted anything for her children but health and happiness. Most of us just don't realize how we're programming our children and the consequences this may have in later life.

Now Matt and I have altered how we speak about illness, injury, and the healing process to Siena. If she wakes up with a tummyache, we remind her that she has the power to heal herself and then often treat her with a placebo—a cough drop or a Tic Tac—or sometimes a dose of cold medicine or a homeopathic remedy. We ask her if she's upset about anything and invite her to talk about her feelings. She's a healthy kid with no significant health issues, so often, this is all she needs. But if that's not enough, when we do give her the pill, we remind her, "This is just to help you feel better *while your body heals itself."*

After we started doing this, she began speaking of illness and injury in a whole new way. She'd fall down and skin her knee, but then she'd jump right up and say, "Don't worry, Mommy. My knee knows how to heal itself."

Siena's father and I have certainly never withheld medical treatment from our child when she needs it—and that's not what I'm suggesting at all. When she fell and split her lip open at three years old, we took her to a surgeon, who gave her general anesthesia so he could repair her lip without causing her too much trauma. If, God forbid, Siena were ever diagnosed with a serious illness, we'd be racing off to the doctor's office lickety-split. But we've found that Siena almost never needs to visit the doctor for anything other than routine checkups. Plus, she now bounces back much more quickly from the cold and flu viruses she brings home from her Waldorf school. Perhaps, when she's older, our childhood programming of her subconscious mind will make it easier for her to overcome any resistance of her mind to the process of self-healing.

But what about you? What if your parents never programmed your subconscious mind to believe it could heal itself? What if you want to believe your mind can heal your body, but you just don't? If you feel hopeless or discouraged, don't despair. The good news is that negative beliefs about health, which trigger nocebo effects and lead to poor health, can be reprogrammed. (For more about how to change subconscious beliefs from disease-inducing beliefs to health-enhancing ones, see Chapter 9.)

Medical Hexing

Once we change our beliefs on a subconscious level, we optimize the culture medium for the community of cells that make up the human body, thereby changing the way our DNA expresses itself. We are not victims of our genes. We are also not masters of our own destiny, completely in control of manifesting what we want and avoiding what we don't want. The truth probably lives somewhere in between. In other words, we have far more power to impact our health than we may realize, but we're also not in charge of life and death (much to the chagrin of the control freak in me.) What we can do is do our best to make the culture medium of our own blood full of the biochemistry of healing rather than the poisonous hormones of chronic, repetitive stress responses.

The data proving that what we believe impacts our physiology was so compelling, yet part of me began to feel irresponsible for not having known about this sooner. When I recited the Hippocratic oath, I had promised to "first, do no harm." I started feeling guilty for any role I might have played in inadvertently harming my patients, both by failing to educate them about how their beliefs could manifest physically and by projecting my own beliefs onto them and possibly hurting them unwittingly.

When we pronounce upon someone with statistics like "Nine out of ten people with your condition die in six months" or "You have a twenty percent chance of five-year survival," is this far from the voodoo practices of some native cultures? Are we cursing them, triggering fear responses in their minds, and causing them to activate stress responses when the body most needs relaxation responses?

When we pronounce our patients "incurable" or even label them with a "chronic" disease like multiple sclerosis or Crohn's disease or high blood pressure, and we tell them they will be afflicted their whole lives, are we not, in essence, harming them? What proof do we have that they will not be one of the health outliers who winds up in the Spontaneous Remission Project, having been cured of a so-called incurable illness?

In *Spontaneous Healing*, Dr. Andrew Weil argues that physicians may unwittingly engage in what he calls "medical hexing." When we pronounce that patients have "chronic," "incurable," or "terminal" illnesses, we may be programming their subconscious minds with negative beliefs and activating stress responses that do more harm than good. By labeling a patient with a negative prognosis and robbing him or her of the hope that cure might be possible, we may ultimately prove the poor prognosis we have bestowed upon our patient correct. Wouldn't we be better off offering hope and triggering the mind to release health-inducing chemicals intended to aid the body's self-repair mechanisms? I'm not suggesting we lie to our patients and offer false hope, but since the truth is that our patients are not statistics, and we are not omniscient psychics who can reliably predict any individual's future, why do we feel the need to curse innocent people with our frightening labels and numbers, all in the name of helping them face "reality"?

When my father was diagnosed with metastatic melanoma, complete with brain and liver metastases, the news was grim. As doctors, Dad and I both knew the stats—less than 5 percent of people with

Dad's condition survived five years, and most died within three to six months.

Looking back and knowing what I now know, I honestly wish we hadn't known those numbers when we found out Dad had melanoma in his brain. With one look at the numbers, hope was dashed—for both of us. We never focused on the 5 percent of people who actually survive. And who's to say Dad couldn't have been one of them? All we could think about was the 95 percent who died—usually very quickly. Dad died right on schedule, exactly three months after his grim diagnosis.

Now, after all I've learned, I realize that doctors who deliver these kinds of numbers to patients may in fact be inadvertently harming their patients. We can't see the future. We have no way to predict which patients will defy the odds and which will succumb quickly. Our intentions are pure. We are motivated by honesty, a commitment to patient autonomy, and the desire to prepare our patients for the worst so they don't wander around in a state of denial.

But if the patient is the one out of ten who doesn't die, have we done him or her any favors by warning of something that might never come to pass? Is our desire for full disclosure worth eliminating hope and shattering beliefs just so our patients can be "realistic" about their prognosis?

I'm not suggesting that we return to the old-school paternalistic model of "Don't worry your pretty little head over it, ma'am." In early 20th-century medicine, doctors would hide a patient's medical condition from the patient because "if Grandma knew, it would just kill her."

Nope. Honesty and collaboration are cornerstones of the doctor-patient relationship and mustn't be tampered with. Education, empowerment, and full disclosure are definitely my modus operandi. But I do question how we deliver the information. Doesn't it make sense for all of us—healers and patients alike—to shift how we think and communicate so we can maximize the body's chance for optimal health?

Some patients calm down when they know statistics. If doctors didn't tell them, they'd look it up on the Internet. Others would prefer to remain blindly optimistic. What if, instead of assuming patients all want to know the statistics of a disease, we ask patients how much they want to know? What if, as patients, we make it clear to our health-care providers when we want to have numbers shared and when we'd prefer to be shielded from those numbers? What if we partner in this way to optimize the chance that some of us may be health outliers, trusting that some wise aspect of our being knows exactly how much we need to know in order to navigate our healing journeys with as much peace as possible.

As a physician, here's what I've learned: somewhere in the intersection of hope, optimism, nurturing care, and full partnership with the empowered patient, a recipe for healing lies.

CHAPTER 3

THE HEALING FACTOR THAT CAN MAKE ALL THE DIFFERENCE

The secret of the care of the patient is in caring for the patient.

— FRANCIS PEABODY

When psychologist Nancy Novack, Ph.D., went to her internist in 2004 with right-sided abdominal pain that she thought was appendicitis, the internist ordered a CT scan and announced that she had stage 4 ovarian cancer, which had metastasized to her liver. Not understanding the severity of her diagnosis, she responded, "Thank goodness it's not appendicitis!" Then, as an afterthought, "What's stage 5?"

She was told she needed to go to surgery—STAT. As soon as an operating room opened, they would perform a "debulking" procedure. Synchronistically, Nancy, a psychologist from the San Francisco Bay Area, was scheduled later that day to meet with a cancer researcher who had his lab near the office where she was waiting for surgery. When she called to reschedule their appointment, the overhead called out "CODE BLUE." The cancer researcher, who could hear the Code Blue in stereo from both the overhead speaker and from his phone, said, "Where are you?"

Nancy told him her scary news and the plan for immediate surgery.

"Do not do anything," the cancer researcher said. "Wait until you hear from me. Do nothing." Nancy felt the urgency of his edict.

Within half an hour, the cancer researcher barged into the internist's office and said to Nancy, "Get your scan. You are going to Stanford. Dr. Brandy Sikic will be waiting for you. MOVE!" The cancer researcher, who had known Dr. Sikic from his medical training, reached the doctor right as he was getting off a plane. He agreed to take on Nancy's case.

Next thing she knew, she was being rushed to Stanford lickety-split. She was swarmed by doctors exploring every bit of her. The surgeons were breathing down her neck, sharpening their scalpels. When Dr. Sikic arrived, he looked at the surgeons and said, "We have no time for surgery. Nancy is too sick for that. We start chemo immediately."

By this time, many of Nancy's family and friends had gathered around her. The doctor, who asked her to call him Brandy, said, "You have a very difficult diagnosis and a challenging prognosis. It will be a rocky road. I believe you can heal. I am with you. When your loved ones go home and you fall apart, I want you to call me. Here is my home phone number."

Nancy gets emotional telling the story. "I called him that night at 2 A.M., and he was as supportive and generous and kind then as he has continued to be for the last 15 years."

After undergoing treatment for a disease with a dismal statistical prognosis, Nancy is happy, cancer free, and committed to the mission statement of her nonprofit "Nancy's List": "Nobody goes through cancer alone."

When I heard Nancy tell me her story, I wanted to bear-hug that doctor. That's what we need: doctors who help us relax our nervous systems and support our bodies to do what they do best—heal. When our nervous systems relax in the presence of health-care providers we trust, any treatment—conventional or otherwise—has a better chance of resulting in a good outcome.

Our trust in modern medicine may even cure us before the doctor walks in! I remember one day when Mom called me, complaining of severe pain in her abdomen. She had been suffering from bloating and bouts of diarrhea since Dad died, but this pain in her belly was new. Mom sounded scared. I reassured her as much as I could from 3,000 miles away.

I scrolled through the differential diagnosis in my mind. Was it her gallbladder? A bleeding ulcer? Pancreatitis? A strange presentation of appendicitis? A bowel obstruction? A hiatal hernia? Reflux?

I peppered her with the requisite questions. Did she have a fever? Had she vomited? When had she last moved her bowels? Was she passing gas? Did she feel hungry?

Her answers led me to believe it was not a surgical emergency. I told her so, but still recommended that she call her primary care doctor. A few minutes later, Mom called me back. She had paged her doctor, and her doctor had asked her to meet her at the office right away.

It was a long drive to the doctor's office—almost an hour. Halfway through the drive, Mom called me, and I asked how she was feeling. The pain had eased a bit. Fifteen minutes later, she had almost arrived at the doctor's office when she called me and said, "Would you believe this darn pain is almost gone?"

By the time she arrived, the pain had disappeared completely.

Mom called me and said, "I swear, this happens to me *all the time*. I want the symptoms to be severe when I get to the doctor's office so they can see me at my worst and help me figure out what's wrong, but more often than not, my symptoms go away before they even call my name."

Bingo.

My mother's doctor never did figure out why she was having the pain, but my conversation with her led me to develop a theory. My mother trusts doctors. She believes they have the power to make her well. Her husband was a doctor, and I became a doctor too. She feels safe when doctors are around. Many times, she has felt poorly, and after seeing doctors, she has felt better. Her mind is now firmly convinced that doctors will help her. And because she chooses her health-care providers carefully, Mom genuinely loves her physicians and feels loved by them in return.

But what if the physical improvement she experiences when she goes to the doctor is primarily the result of her mind and its effect on her perception of her symptoms? When Mom calls the doctor and makes an appointment, what if her mind registers relaxation, hope, optimism, tenderness, and the belief that healing is on the way? Her brain lets out a huge sigh of relief. Her thoughts shut down the stress responses she experienced when she first noticed the pain, the idea of visiting the doctor elicits a relaxation response, the body rests, her body is filled with natural endorphins and other healing hormones, and her self-repair mechanisms get activated. Before she knows it, the body has taken care of the problem, and voilà! The symptoms are gone.

The trip to the doctor winds up getting all the credit, but the real hero is her own mind and the biochemistry of healing it elicits.

Of course, this is not to diminish what doctors can do. When my then husband Matt cut two fingers off his hand with a table saw, and his doctor, Dr. Jonathan Jones, stitched them back on with advanced microsurgical techniques, Matt and I were in full-on worship mode. This brilliant man, who came in on his day off, used a microscope to sew back together every artery, nerve, and bone in Matt's fingers so Matt, an artist and a writer, could still use his hands. I was so grateful to my physician colleague that I made him a painting of my own hand as a gesture of my respect for the skill, love, commitment, and devotion he had shown to Matt.

But as much as I'm grateful to Dr. Jones, I credit Matt with much of his recovery. From the get-go, Matt held a belief that his fingers would be sewed back on and work as well as they had before he lost them. He had perfect faith in modern medicine, and even after cutting his fingers off, he looked at me with wide eyes and said, "It's all going to be okay." He felt no pain during the incident, probably because his body was full of pain-relieving endorphins, and when I called 911 and the paramedics arrived, Matt expressed relief. I can only imagine that his brain was spitting out healing hormones and health-inducing chemicals that aided his recovery and made Dr. Jones's job easier.

The truth of the matter is that someone still had to sew those fingers back on. I've heard hard-to-believe stories about healers who spontaneously repaired fractures and closed cuts without sutures or scars, but chances are good that those fingers weren't going to replant themselves. The mind-body-spirit connection is a powerful tool for healing, but it has its limits. That said, when the surgeon cuts out a tumor or prescribes an antibiotic or sets a broken bone, we still depend on the body's self-repair mechanisms to finish the job. Matt's body still had to fuse those reconnected bones and heal those cuts in his arteries and nerves. Dr. Jones made it possible for his body to do so, but his body had to do the rest. The rejection rate of replanted limbs and digits is high. While Dr. Jones gets much of the credit, Matt's unshakable faith in modern medicine and his relaxed, trusting mind-set in the face of disaster may have made all the difference.

I want to make it clear that, when I talk about the body's ability to repair itself, I am *in no way* suggesting that we should forego the advances modern medicine now makes available to us. While I believe our bodies have a remarkable capacity for self-repair, I also believe we shouldn't expect our bodies to do all the heavy lifting, and sometimes, the body will simply fail if we expect it to do all the work. Modern medical technology has performed at least as many and probably more miracles than the stories we hear on the Internet about patients healing themselves or healers treating "incurable" illnesses. If you had told someone a hundred years ago that someone who cut off his limb might get it successfully sewed back on, or a child whose heart stopped working might get a new heart, they would have called such procedures miracles. Miracles are in the eye of the beholder, and personally, I prefer to see all radical cures as miracles, regardless of how the miracle came about.

While my mother might not have needed her doctor's touch to cure her belly pain, Matt clearly needed Dr. Jones. Sometimes we rely on the technology modern medicine has to offer, and sometimes we don't. But I can promise you this: in either scenario, finding the right person to support your healing journey is crucial, and the scientific data I studied confirms this.

The Doctor as Medicine

Patients get well, at least in part, because they believe in the power of modern medicine and expect to feel relief when they see doctors and other health-care specialists they trust. My mother and Matt are not alone in placing great faith and trust in doctors. Many people experience similar conditioned responses when visiting the doctor. Patients become accustomed to going to the doctor and subsequently feeling better, so the mind may work its magic before the therapeutic encounter has actually happened, even with no direct therapeutic intervention.

But what does the scientific data show?

I went back to the medical journals, and from what I learned, a nurturing therapeutic relationship may be responsible for a large part of the positive response patients experience when treated with placebos. Scientists postulate that it wouldn't be enough to just imbibe placebos if they were self-administered without the participation of a physician—that to be truly powerful, someone in whom the patient places great faith must deliver them.

In an interview on NPR, placebo researcher Ted Kaptchuk said, "A sugar pill doesn't do anything. What does something is the context of healing. It's the rituals healing. It's being in a healing relationship. . . . But the placebo pill is a wonderful tool, or a saline injection is a wonderful tool, to isolate what is usually in the background, take it away from the medications and procedures that medicine does, and actually study just the act of caring. That's, I think, what we're measuring when we study placebo effects."[1]

When Kaptchuk, who is trained as a Chinese medicine practitioner and acupuncturist, was asked how he, as a scientist, justified practicing acupuncture when most randomized, controlled clinical trials failed to demonstrate its effectiveness beyond placebo, he said, "Because I am a damn good healer. That is the difficult truth. If you needed help and you came to me, you would get better. Thousands of people have. Because, in the end, it isn't really about the needles. It's about the man."[2]

Kaptchuk's sentiments are affirmed in the *New England Journal of Medicine* article he co-wrote, which studied asthmatics. Those who reported being short of breath were treated with an albuterol inhaler (standard treatment for asthma), a sham inhaler (placebo), fake acupuncture (also placebo), and no treatment. All of the treated patients felt equally better—approximately 50 percent improvement for those treated with albuterol, the sham inhaler, and the fake acupuncture, compared to a 21 percent improvement in those receiving no treatment.

However, unlike other studies, which demonstrated physiological responses that coincided with symptomatic relief, when researchers in this study measured lung function in the asthmatics, the physiological response did not equal the patient's subjective experience. Those who received fake acupuncture, a sham inhaler, and no treatment all experienced improved lung function (7 percent) but not nearly as much as those getting albuterol (20 percent).[3]

Why were these asthmatics feeling better, even when their bodies weren't demonstrating physiological responses to explain the clinical improvement? Perhaps patients in the study were feeling better, not just because of the albuterol, fake acupuncture, or sham inhaler, but because *somebody cared*. What if the patients were treated not by the medicine itself but by the medical care? Perhaps the treatment groups felt equally better because they received equal care, and perhaps that's even more important than the drug or treatment they receive.

Asthma may be different from cancer. When you're battling a life-threatening illness, it's not so much the symptom relief you're after; it's the disease remission. Is the cancer gone or not? But what if symptom relief and disease remission are linked by the therapeutic experience and its relationship to the mind, the damages of the stress response, and the healing power of the relaxation response?

I suspected there was a potent link, but once again, I wanted proof.

Proof That Nurturing Care Makes a Difference

At this point in my research, I strongly suspected that a huge part of the placebo effect revolved around the delivery of nurturing care and the therapeutic rituals of medicine. I had a sneaking suspicion that lack of loving care—especially with regard to medical hexing—could elicit nocebo effects. But how much of an effect did it have, and was there any evidence that the bedside manner or beliefs of the health-care provider affected health outcomes?

Dr. Lawrence Egbert conducted a study at Harvard Medical School, published in the *New England Journal of Medicine*, for which he randomized preoperative surgical patients into two groups. One group met with cheerful, optimistic anesthesiologists who assured them that their surgery was going to be a piece of cake, they were going to be comfortable and pain free, and everything was going to be peachy. The other, unfortunate patients (poor babies!) were attended by anesthesiologists instructed to be grumpy, rushed, and unsympathetic. (Interestingly, they were actually the same anesthesiologists wearing two different hats.) Those who got the optimistic anesthesiologists required only half the amount of painkilling medication and were discharged an average of 2.6 days earlier.[4]

Optimism on the part of the physician also makes a difference. Fueled by the comment "The reason why Dr. Smith is so successful is because he's so positive," in 1987, Dr. K. B. Thomas was inspired to conduct a study on whether a physician's positive attitude affects patient outcomes. His study, conducted at the University of Southampton and published in the *British Medical Journal*, evaluated 200 of his own patients who didn't feel well but didn't have any apparent abnormalities on examination. The patients were randomly selected to receive one of four different types of consultations: a consultation conducted in a "positive manner," with and without treatment, and a consultation conducted in a "non-positive manner," with and without treatment. Sixty-four percent of those receiving a positive consultation got better, compared with 39 percent of those who received a negative consultation. The study found that patient recovery could be increased by words that suggested the patient "would be better in a few days" and, if he was given treatment, that "the treatment would certainly make him better." On the flip side, negative words such as "I am not sure that the treatment I am going to give you will have an effect" led to longer recovery times.[5] Thomas concluded, "The doctor himself is a powerful therapeutic agent; he is the placebo and his influence is felt to a greater or lesser extent at every consultation."[6]

While optimism and positive words are key, trust is just as important. Nocebo effects can occur when a patient distrusts medical personnel and the therapies they implement.[7] I used to work in a public health clinic in San Diego, where most of my patients were Somali refugees. Coming from a culture where medicine is practiced much differently, many of my patients were deeply distrusting of American doctors and the treatments we prescribed. In this patient population, I witnessed far more side effects resulting from common, seemingly innocuous treatments, such as prenatal vitamins, than my American patients usually reported. Although I worked hard to earn the trust of these patients, I suspect these side effects occurred because some of them genuinely believed we were trying to poison them.

What your doctor believes also matters. In a study published in *The Lancet*, which investigated the role of endorphins in how placebos relieve pain, researchers found that, despite the use of a double-blind procedure, the expectations of the physicians still influenced how patients responded to injections of fentanyl, naloxone, or placebo.[8] If the doctor doesn't believe a certain treatment will work, the treatment may actually be less effective.

Another study conducted by the National Institute of Mental Health assessed 250 depressed patients, who were randomized into four 16-week treatment groups: interpersonal psychotherapy, cognitive behavior therapy, the antidepressant imipramine, and placebo. As a substudy of the larger project, researchers at Georgetown videotaped how doctors participating in this study interacted with patients and, based on these video exchanges, asked expert raters to predict who would get well and who wouldn't.

Surprisingly, these raters were able to predict this, based on the doctor-patient relationship, regardless of which treatment the patient was given. It wasn't just whether or not the doctor and patient connected emotionally. What the doctor believed about the patient's prognosis also turned out to be crucial. If a doctor believed that the patient would improve, he or she was more likely to do so than if the doctor did not radiate this type of positivity.[9] These findings about physician beliefs have since been replicated in many other studies, not just in the field of mental health but also in other areas.

Not surprisingly, the personality of the physician makes a difference as well. A Harvard Medical School study published in the *British Medical Journal* demonstrated that the response to a placebo increased from 44 percent to 62 percent when the doctor treated the patient with "warmth, attention, and confidence." Among a third control group of people on a waiting list who received no medical care at all, only 28 percent improved.[10]

The right support, combined with positive belief, can even result in inexplicable cure. In the early 1950s, Dr. Albert Mason at the Queen Victoria Hospital in West Sussex, England, treated a teenage boy with thick, cracked, leathery skin covering most of his body. His condition was believed to be a severe case of warts, and since hypnosis had previously been described as an effective treatment for warts, Dr. Mason genuinely believed hypnosis could cure the warts, even at such an advanced stage.[11]

Convinced of the mind's power to induce self-repair of warts, Dr. Mason got to work. During the first session, Dr. Mason focused solely on the boy's arm, bringing the boy into a trance state and guiding him through the process of seeing his arm as pink and healthy. After repeated treatment, the skin was nearly normal, to the shock and awe of Dr. Mason's peers. But Dr. Mason wasn't surprised. He had faith that the mind could heal the body, at least for a condition like severe warts.

When the boy was then seen by his surgeon, who had unsuccessfully tried to help the boy with skin grafts, the surgeon was amazed to see the boy's healthy skin, especially because the surgeon had made a mistake. Instead of suffering from warts, the boy had been misdiagnosed. His real condition was a severe, potentially lethal genetic condition called congenital ichthyosis.

Although no evidence had ever demonstrated that the mind could cure congenital ichthyosis, both Dr. Mason and the boy had believed hypnosis would work. And it did.

Word got out, and others who suffered from congenital ichthyosis sought out Dr. Mason, who tried to help them. But Dr. Mason was unable to later replicate the same effect in others. He blamed his failure on his own lack of belief. While he believed hypnosis would cure warts, he doubted its efficacy for this more serious genetic condition, even though hypnosis had already cured it once.

The Ritual of Medicine

A sugar pill, while powerful, is really just a sugar pill. It's not magic. While some treatments, like my husband's hand surgery, repair the body in ways the body could not induce alone, other treatments merely enlist the potent power of your consciousness to optimize the health of the body, and the support of a caring health-care provider makes all the difference.

Some studies—like K. B. Thomas's—go so far as to suggest that the doctor is, in fact, the placebo, that the role the physician plays, in and of itself, triggers the self-healing response.[12] What we've learned from the placebo effect is that, as Ted Kaptchuk explains, the placebo strips away the actual treatments we assume cure us—the antibiotics, the knee surgery, the antidepressants, the painkillers, the chest surgery—distilling medicine down to something therapeutic that has less to do with pills or surgery and more to do with love. Without the biochemical trappings of medicine, we're left only with medicine as it used to be back before highly effective treatments like Matt's finger surgery existed—the ritual of medicine, the meaning we ascribe to the medical treatment, and the care of someone devoted to trying to help us get well.

Because the role of the physician in the Western world has been imbued with so much meaning in our modern culture, the support of a caring physician may carry even more weight than the same kind of support from a pastor, therapist, acupuncturist, or other loving, healing presence. Yet the same might not be true in other cultures, where the greatest healing power may lie with the shaman, the Chinese medicine doctor, or the medicine woman. As reported in *The New York Times*,[13] one California hospital that catered to Hmong immigrants from northern Laos instituted a policy to allow Hmong shamans into the hospital with the same unrestricted access as doctors or clergy. As Hmong shaman Va Meng Lee said, "Doctors are good at disease. The soul is the shaman's responsibility." Because Hmong culture places a great deal of weight on the role of the shaman, it strikes me as good medicine to allow indigenous healers to collaborate with doctors to attend to healing ceremonies and rituals most doctors do not perform. If the ritual of medicine is a foundational part of the healing process, we need to be sensitive to the cultural beliefs of patients in order to maximize the benefits of this aspect of the therapeutic experience.

One doctor I interviewed—we'll call her Dr. M—said, "I know that the most valuable thing I offer my patients is love." She told me a story about a patient with severe nerve pain that plagued 90 percent of her body. The patient had seen dozens of physicians and quite a few alternative medicine healers, without relief. Then she saw Dr. M, who prescribed fish oil and B vitamins. Dr. M admitted to me that she prescribed the supplements mostly as a placebo, because there was no clinical evidence to support the idea that they would be effective against this nerve pain. She also spent hours listening to this patient and offering her nurturing care.

Soon afterward, the patient fell head over heels in love with a young man, and shortly thereafter, she returned to Dr. M's office to announce that her pain was gone. She credited the B vitamins and fish oil, calling them a miracle cure.

But Dr. M told me, "I knew it wasn't the vitamins. I believe it was the love of this young man—in combination with the care I offered—that cured her."

The Mechanism of Nurturing Care

How can the nurturing care, positive belief, and state of consciousness of a health-care provider result in better health of the patient? Scientists don't fully understand the mechanisms of this process, but it's likely that it all goes back to the illness-inducing stress response and the self-repair-facilitating relaxation response. When a patient who imbues the physician with positive meaning feels tended, trusting, reassured, and nurtured, the stress response is aborted. The relaxation response is induced. Perhaps the patient is even entrained into a higher level of consciousness by an exceptionally calm, loving, supportive health-care provider. Imagine how that feels for someone who is scared, in pain, and sick. With the body's self-repair mechanisms flipped back on, the patient starts to get better right away.

Just imagine you're diagnosed with cancer, as Nancy was when she was told she had stage 4 ovarian cancer. The minute you hear the word *cancer*, your fight-or-flight stress responses go crazy. The adrenal gland pumps out cortisol. The sympathetic nervous system jumps to attention. The word *cancer* is interpreted by the mind as a deadly threat, even though the threat of death isn't usually imminent at the time of diagnosis. In such a state of physiological stress, the body is poorly equipped to fight cancer. It's too busy preparing to fight and flee.

Then in walks the oncologist, who is like Nancy's doctor—kind, nurturing, and reassuring. He holds your hand, hugs you when you cry, and assures you that he has cared for thousands of people with just such a cancer, and most of them have done well. With calm words and gentle presence, the oncologist explains that no matter what happens, you will never be alone, that he will be right there by your side, doing everything in his power to help. With your input and sensitivity to your preferences, beliefs, spirituality, and worldview, a treatment plan is made, and he gives you a phone number you can call if you think of any more questions. He offers you another hug or a gentle pat on the back. Even though you're facing a big surgery and months of chemotherapy, you feel better already.

Why? Because the mind is soothed. The fear is alleviated. The stress response is turned off. The body relaxes. The doctor has convinced your brain that all will be well, or at least that everything will be done to try to ensure that it will be. In such a relaxed state, the body can get busy doing what it does best—making efforts to heal itself.

The Absence of Nurturing Care Can Harm You

So if calming, reassuring doctors who believe all will be well can induce such positive physiological effects, we know what happens when physicians unwittingly use their superpowers in the wrong way. Although they may mean well, all too often, doctors and other health-care providers not only fail to treat their patients with nurturing care and tenderness; they may even allow themselves to get so busy, overworked, and depleted that they flat-out harm their patients.

A friend wrote to me after leaving her doctor's office:

> *Lissa, if this doctor robs me as I leave the building, I won't be able to confirm it was him, as I don't think he looked at me once. From the nurse intake to the actual exam room, both practitioners faced AWAY from me, toward their computer terminals, while they asked me questions and clicked away at the keyboard. The computer fed him my new prescription, and he never even discussed it with me. If a computer program is all I need to monitor and refill prescriptions on my current or chronic conditions, then what am I doing spending an hour in a waiting room, waiting to look at some guy's back? Oh, and don't forget—the nurse clearly put a wrong code into the computer, because he came in prepared to give me a BREAST exam, rather than listening to my asthmatic CHEST. I was like, "What are you talking about, sir? You have the wrong information, or else the wrong room." Sigh. I'm so mad right now. I'm never coming here ever again.*

I've heard this kind of feedback frequently from my online community. With many health-care providers feeling overburdened, exhausted, and unappreciated, patients sometimes wind up feeling more stressed after a doctor's visit than they did before. If you have to sit for two hours in a crowded waiting room, only to have seven and a half minutes with an exhausted doctor who cuts you off, forgets your name, never lays a hand on you, and then scares you with a disconcerting prognosis, you can be sure your stress responses will be activated.

Nobody intends for this to happen, but sometimes it does. The reality is that you need to trust your health-care providers, yet the devastating truth is that, at least in the United States, the current health-care system has become inherently hard to trust because, although intentions are good and lip service is given to patient well-being, the financial bottom line has surpassed nurturing patient care as the number one priority. This violates the intentions of the dedicated people who work within the system, the ones who enter into the practice of medicine, nursing, and other health-care fields in order to be someone patients can trust when they are at their most vulnerable. If you were to ask doctors, nurses, and other health-care practitioners to redesign the health-care system, we would have a very different system. The system is failing, not only for patients in clinics and hospitals, but for all those who serve within these systems and experience daily the conflict between the demands of the system, the regulation of individual practice, and the wish to do no harm.

Health-care providers have often sacrificed so much for their patients that they lose touch with why they're doing what they were called to do. They think the sacrifices they've made demonstrate the care they have for their patients. But sacrifices are not enough. It's time to put the *care* back in health care. Doctors and other health-care providers need to remember why we do what we do so we can maximize the healing effect we have on our patients, especially when things go wrong. The need to restore the heart and soul of medicine fueled me to found the Whole Health Medicine Institute, a consciousness and healing training program for health-care providers and those who long to be true healers. It educates doctors and others in the medical field about the Six Steps to Healing Yourself from this book, as well as exposes them to over 30 faculty members who are pioneers in mind-body medicine, energy healing, psycho-spiritual healing, indigenous medicine, trauma healing, and other healing modalities not commonly taught in medical schools. Part of this education explores how best to be a healing presence that optimally supports our patients on their healing journeys, which includes "heal the healer" work aimed at healing the traumas many doctors face in the process of becoming experts. As long as we are wounded healers blended with our wounds, we cannot show up with the grounded, embodied, intuitive, loving presence that helps people heal. (Learn more or enroll in the Whole Health Medicine Institute at http://wholehealthmedicineinstitute.com.)

How to Deliver Bad News

In 1974, Dr. Clifton Meador told his patient Sam Londe, who suffered from cancer of the esophagus, that his condition was considered fatal. After Dr. Meador broke the news about his death sentence, Sam died quickly, only weeks after his diagnosis.

But an autopsy performed after his death surprised doctors. Very little cancer was found—certainly not enough to kill him. Dr. Meador told the Discovery Health Channel, "He died with cancer, but not from cancer." Why did he die? Perhaps the bad news triggered so much fear that stress responses wreaked havoc in his body. He died because he was told he would die and he *believed* he would die. His negative thoughts translated into real physiological changes. As I detail in my book *The Fear Cure: Cultivating Courage as Medicine for the Body, Mind, and Soul*, shock and fear can literally scare you to an instantaneous death in the absence of underlying disease.

Decades later, Sam Londe's death still haunts Dr. Meador, who said, "I thought he had cancer. He thought he had cancer. Everybody around him thought he had cancer. Did I remove hope in some way?"[14]

I suspect that this kind of thing is not uncommon. Of course, doctors never mean to harm patients. Most are motivated by the purest intentions, and we want nothing more than to help our patients heal. But I've heard good doctors give the bad news spiel time and time again. It often goes something like this:

Door #1

I'm afraid your cancer is inoperable and is not limited to the one organ we thought it was. In fact, it's in your stomach, your colon, your lymph nodes, and dotted all over the lining of your abdomen. We haven't done the studies yet, but it may also be in your lungs, your bones, and your brain.

If you'd like, we can give you chemotherapy, but it will just be palliative, not curative. I'm very sorry to give you this news, and of course, we'll do everything we can to keep you comfortable. But this would be a good time to get your affairs in order. If you haven't updated your will, you might want to do that, because only 1 in 20 people with your kind of cancer survive five years, and most die within three to six months.

I'm terribly sorry to have to tell you this, and of course, we can talk further when the effects of the anesthesia have worn off and you're a little more awake.

When bad news is delivered this way, it only triggers stress responses that make it harder for the patient's body to repair itself and, in rare cases, may even lead to death when there is no apparent cause. It's possible that you really can be scared to death.

I propose a new way to deliver bad news. Let's take the same patient we described behind Door #1—the one with metastatic cancer and a 1-in-20 chance of survival. Let's give her some time to wake up from her anesthesia. Let's comfort her in the recovery room. Let's tell the family we'll have a family conference when she fully wakes up, and then let's have this conversation, which we script for our students at the Whole Health Medicine Institute:

Door #2

I have good news and bad news, so I'll get the bad news out of the way first. I'm afraid the cancer isn't limited to one organ, the way we had hoped it would be. [Pause for a moment to give this time to sink in.]

The cancer also appears to have spread to your stomach, your colon, your lymph nodes, and the lining of your abdomen. We'll have to do some tests to see if the cancer might have spread anywhere else, and we should be able to get that information very soon so we can make a plan about what's next. But I want you to know you will not go through this alone. [Pause again.]

I know that's a lot to hear right now, but let me share with you the good news. The good news is that a percentage of people with exactly this diagnosis survive, and there are some predictors of who those people might be. The body is designed to repair itself when it gets sick, and we have clear evidence that those who nurture their bodies, minds, and spirits while staying hopeful and believing in their ability to get well are more likely to be cured. It's important to your body that we all remain optimistic and that your mind and body stay as relaxed as possible, because only in this state of relaxation can your body fight off the cancer.

I want you to know that I believe that it's possible for you to be cured from this cancer, and I will be here to support you every step of the way. We'll talk tomorrow about treatment options and where we can go from here, but why don't you get some rest first and spend some time processing this with your family. Before I go to do my next surgery, do you have any questions for me right now? [Pause and listen.]

I'll talk to you again first thing in the morning, and if you have any urgent questions that come up between now and then, feel free to give me a call. Here's my number in case you need me. I know this isn't the news you wanted to hear today, but please, never give up hope. I believe in miracles, and you just might be that miracle.

Imagine how differently you would feel after each conversation. The first doctor would likely leave you feeling stressed, uncertain, and upset. The doctor behind Door #2, however, would probably make you feel supported, hopeful, and well informed, so much so that your mind and body are relaxed.

I think it's our responsibility as health-care providers to consider how we might facilitate the process of helping our patients hold realistic but healing beliefs and release hopeless, disease-inducing ones so we can limit stress responses and elicit relaxation responses that help the body heal itself and prevent further damage. Perhaps this act of love and service will have more profound effects than any drug or surgery. It may take a few more minutes out of our day to deliver bad news in a way that facilitates healing, but the results could be extraordinary.

Physician, Heal Thyself

When health-care professionals hold space with nurturing care, we create the ideal environment for patients to heal themselves. But all too often, we make the mistake of trying to serve those in need of healing from a place of depletion. As doctors, we are taught to sacrifice our own needs in order to serve others. We wind up severely sleep-deprived, we eat poorly, we fail to tend to our relationships, we neglect our self-care, we close our hearts to protect ourselves from all the trauma we witness and experience, and we often wind up physically, emotionally, and spiritually unhealthy. The minute a doctor or other health-care provider gives to the point of depletion, the well is dry, and although we still have our expertise, we deprive our patients of the additional gift of healing presence. Because we are so depleted, we feel victimized, and we wind up becoming the villains, lashing out at patients because we are running on empty.

If I could wave a magic wand and change one thing about the health-care system, I would change the insane notion that, in order to be good health-care providers, we must give at the expense of our own health. It's impossible to be fully present for our patients, to open our hearts as widely as they must be opened, and to serve as fully as we can when we have nothing left to give. If only doctors could be models of self-care so that patients might learn by example, the whole system would undergo a radical shift. If healers could heal themselves first, we would be able to serve and love from a place of wholeness so we could more effectively heal the world.

15 Ways Healers Can Amplify Their Art

1. Listen.

2. Open your heart.

3. Take your hand off the doorknob, sit down, turn your back to the computer, face the patient, and make eye contact.

4. Be present.

5. Offer safe, healing touch.

6. Invite your patient to be your partner.

7. Avoid judgment.

8. Educate, but don't dictate.

9. Choose your words with care, and remain realistically optimistic.

10. Trust your patient's intuition.

11. Be respectful of other practitioners who are treating your patient.

12. Reassure your patients they are not alone.

13. Encourage stress relief and let your presence relieve stress.

14. Be a merchant of hope, because no matter how grim the prognosis, spontaneous remission is always possible.

15. Set the intention that healing may happen, then let go.

Healing yourself is hard work, and nobody should have to do it alone. As physicians, we can dose up life-saving treatment, but if we fail to heal ourselves so that we are full enough to sprinkle our treatments with a heaping helping of love, we limit the ability of our patients to fully and sustainably recover.

Norman Cousins, author of *Anatomy of an Illness*, knows this well. Cousins had been diagnosed with the degenerative collagen disorder ankylosing spondylitis, and he believed he would be able to arrest his condition if he were discharged from the hospital and treated with high doses of vitamin C and daily laughter instead of anti-inflammatory drugs, painkillers, and tranquilizers. Fortunately, his doctor, with whom Cousins enjoyed a collaborative partnership based on mutual respect, supported his decision.

In *Anatomy of an Illness*, Cousins wrote, "I would say that the principal contribution made by my doctor to the taming, and possibly the conquest, of my illness was that he encouraged me to believe I was a respected partner with him in the total undertaking."

The Placebo Effect in Complementary and Alternative Medicine

Perhaps nurturing care, presence, and the consciousness of the healer explain why many patients experience remarkable results when treated by complementary and alternative medicine (CAM) treatments, which include such therapies as acupuncture, Chinese medicine, homeopathy, herbal medicine, energy medicine, craniosacral therapy, chiropractic medicine, shamanism, and other such modalities. Many CAM treatments fail to demonstrate clinically relevant and statistically significant benefits when compared to placebo, but this could be because modern science doesn't yet have a way to test for or provide an adequate placebo control for the consciousness of the healer. Science assumes that the treatment itself is the most relevant intervention. But perhaps the intervention is far less important than the person providing the intervention. As Kaptchuk stated earlier with regard to his acupuncture practice, it isn't "about the needles." Whether we're talking about hands-on healing, herbs, acupuncture needles, or conventional chemotherapy, perhaps we're thinking about this all wrong. Maybe the one providing the intervention has far more to do with the healing process than whatever treatment they think provides the healing.

Please understand, I'm not writing off all modern medicine or CAM interventions as "all placebo." I'm only proposing that practitioners may have far more to do with helping patients facilitate optimal outcomes than just the treatment they offer. In other words, we think it's the treatment—the drug, the surgery, the herb, or the energy healing—that's curing the patient. And perhaps this is true. Certainly, in the instance of Matt's amputated fingers, I believe the success of his outcome was the direct result of Dr. Jones's exceptional microsurgical talents. But I also believe that his loving presence and his calm, confident certainty that Matt's hand would be restored to full function also participated in helping Matt's finger replants "take." So, yes, it's worthwhile to use science to prove whether interventions are indeed effective. Such science has evolved us beyond the charlatans of snake-oil days. But separating the practitioner from the intervention in scientific studies may be harder than researchers understand.

In the seven years since I first published *Mind Over Medicine*, I've globe-trotted around the world on a quest to unravel the mysteries of miraculous healing, working with shamans in the Andes of Peru, qigong masters from China, Balinese healers, and spiritual healers, energy healers, and biofield researchers in the United States. I now believe it's impossible to fully separate the treatment from the one doing the treating. I also believe that practitioners can be an essential part of the sorts of miracle cures patients and healers worldwide report.

In *Anatomy of an Illness*, Norman Cousins wrote, "The vaunted 'miracle cures' that abound in the literature of all the great religions all say something about the ability of the patient, properly motivated and stimulated, to participate actively in extraordinary reversals of disease and disability." Perhaps it is the role of the practitioner to properly motivate, stimulate, and, I would add, relax the patient's nervous system so the natural, everyday bodily process of healing can resume.

In an editorial in the *British Medical Journal*, Yale professor Dr. David Spiegel chided skeptics of CAM healing methods for implying that, if most of the benefit of CAM therapies comes from the placebo effect, they should be consigned to the realm of quackery. He posed this question: "Is it possible that the alternative medical community has tended historically to understand something important about the experience of illness and the ritual of doctor-patient interactions that the rest of medicine might do well to hear?"[15]

Our reductionist medical model wants us to believe that any doctor who administers the same drug should get the same result from the patient, but whether we're talking about CAM practitioners or doctors, what I can say with as much certainty as this kind of inquiry allows me is that the one who provides whatever treatment your intuition guides you to seek out is of tantamount importance. So choose wisely.

Reclaiming the Heart of Medicine

As health-care providers, we are blessed with a sacred opportunity. We have the power to encourage relaxation responses in our patients and, in so doing, be part of the healing process in more ways than just drugs or surgeries. In my opinion, if we fail to optimize the self-healing mechanisms of our patients, we do them—and ourselves—a huge disservice. And if we step up to the plate and do our job well, our role in the healing process may mean the difference between life and death for the patient.

I often joke that I practice love, with a little medicine on the side. Yet, all too often, technological advances have so distanced us from our patients that the love seems to have gotten lost in the process. Whereas a physician used to do house calls, sit at the bedside, and touch the patient, we now offer 13-minute patient visits in a sterile white room where lab tests may take the place of a thorough patient history and radiologic studies may even replace the hands-on physical exam. Without the healing power of listening, loving touch, nurturing care, and healing intention, what are we offering patients beyond straight technology?

When you're facing a health crisis, make sure you find the nurturing care you need. It's not enough to seek out the most technically skilled surgeon or the most famous university doctor who specializes in your specific illness. Though specialized skills certainly come in handy, if you want to optimize your body's chance of cure, you'll also want to ensure that your health-care providers genuinely offer you a healing presence. You may need more than just one person as you navigate the course of your treatment. You may need a whole team believing in you, offering you tools from their various toolboxes, and helping you make the body ripe for miracles. As you gather your team, you'll also need the members of that team to cooperate with one another.

Acupuncturist Susan Fox calls such a team of collaborative practitioners "the healing round table." The healing round table is a collaborative process in which all health-care practitioners involved in the care of the patient are equal players whose opinions matter. At the healing round table, the patient, not the doctor, presides as the utmost authority. While physicians might be invited to the healing round table, the invitation to be present does not grant doctors the right to give orders, negate the advice of others, disrespect others at the table, or, most importantly, disregard the patient's wishes.

While I understand the need to have a physician calling out orders during a trauma situation in the emergency room, the same does not apply to those caring for someone with a chronic illness. I once heard a respected physician (albeit a tired one) say to a brilliant nurse, "Let's play a little game. I'll play doctor. You play nurse. I'll give the orders, and you *follow them.*" This kind of power trip serves neither the health-care provider nor the patient.

I've also heard doctors ridicule patients for seeking out CAM treatments, disrespecting both the patient and the CAM practitioner. These kinds of adversarial relationships trouble me deeply, because they speak to a much greater dysfunction within our health-care system. This dictatorial, condescending, hierarchical, power-tripping mind-set is more militaristic than the way I believe health-care systems should be. And while doctors in the trenches may feel they are at war against disease, replicating warlike methods of communication within hospitals and patient exam rooms doesn't help people heal. It only triggers stress responses. Health care functions much more effectively when teams work as a unit committed to serving the patient first and foremost, without ego, competition, and unnecessary power plays.

With the practitioners I've been training at the Whole Health Medicine Institute, I've been recruiting health-care revolutionaries—health-care providers who are committed to bringing the *care* back to health care. But health-care providers can't do this alone. We need YOU too. The good news is that our numbers are growing, and we *will* revolutionize health care, not by competing with the current system or going to war with it, but by expanding to include it alongside other tools in the medical toolbox. As mind-body medicine pioneer Dr. Larry Dossey wrote to me, "We really do constitute a kind of parallel medical world that exists alongside the conventional kind. We focus on what [the conventional world] knows, and we honor it, but more besides: spirituality, meaning, purpose, consciousness, compassion, empathy, love . . ."

We're here, an increasingly organized and vocal population of change agents who know we must reclaim the heart of medicine and are committed to seeing change happen. I know you may feel discouraged, but keep the faith. It takes a village, and we need you now more than ever.

The time is now. Are you ready?

PART TWO

TREAT YOUR MIND

CHAPTER 4

THE WHOLE HEALTH CAIRN

The great majority of us are required to live a life of constant, systematic duplicity. Your health is bound to be affected if, day after day, you say the opposite of what you feel, if you grovel before what you dislike and rejoice at what brings you nothing but misfortune. Our nervous system isn't just a fiction, it's part of our physical body, and our soul exists in space and is inside us, like teeth in our mouth. It can't be forever violated with impunity.

— BORIS PASTERNAK, *DOCTOR ZHIVAGO*

Like many of my patients in my Marin Country practice, Marla obsessively cared for her body in all the ways people in the multibillion-dollar wellness industry recommend. She ate a vegetarian diet, hiked and practiced yoga, competed in triathlons, took dozens of supplements her naturopath had given her, and avoided alcohol, smoking, and using any illegal drugs.

But she had a medical chart two feet thick and suffered from four different chronic health conditions.

Marla had heard from some friends that my practice wasn't your usual medical practice, so she scheduled an appointment with me to see if I could figure out why she was still sick in spite of all of her efforts to get well. From reading the new patient intake probing into Marla's personal life, I found out that she was miserable. She was in a physically and mentally abusive marriage and hadn't had sex in two years. She felt creatively thwarted because her husband didn't support her passion for art, and she was so busy at work and training for races, she didn't make time to paint. Plus, she was exhausted from caring for her aging, sick mother, who lived in her home.

After I finished reading her form, I knew that Marla's body was never going to get well until she healed these other aspects of her life. With all those negative emotions filling her mind and all those stress hormones coursing through her body, no vegetable, supplement, exercise program, or drug was going to be strong enough to counteract the harmful health effects of chronic stress responses on her body.

After sharing with Marla my thoughts about the real reason her body was suffering, I asked her the big question: "What does your body need in order to heal?"

Marla said, "I need to move to Santa Fe."

"Why Santa Fe?" I asked.

Marla said, "I have a vacation home in Santa Fe, and whenever I go there, *all of my symptoms disappear.*"

Perhaps there was a biochemical explanation for this. Maybe she had some chemical sensitivity to something in her Mill Valley house. Maybe she was allergic to something that grew in the Bay Area but not in Santa Fe. Perhaps the weather or the food or some other environmental factor could explain such a dramatic difference.

But I doubted it, so I encouraged Marla to listen to the wisdom of her body and her intuition.

A year later, I got a call from Marla telling me she had moved to Santa Fe. In order to make such a drastic move, she sold her company and helped her mother establish herself in a wonderful retirement community close to Santa Fe, where she would be able to visit her on weekends. She also filed for divorce from her husband. And once Marla got to Santa Fe, she enrolled in art school. She had since fallen in love with a new man and met a whole new group of artist friends, and she enjoyed hiking, biking, and skiing in the mountains outside of Santa Fe.

Most importantly, she told me, all of her symptoms had disappeared, as if by magic, within three months of her move.

Marla's health conditions were not cured by a drug, supplement, or surgery, but by reducing the stress in her life, relaxing her mind and body, following a dream, finding love, and filling her body with health-inducing hormones while ridding it of harmful stress hormones. I found out later that Marla also started working with an indigenous healer in Santa Fe who facilitated her through a lot of trauma release and soul retrieval work. Such changes resulted in measurable physiological changes in her body.

And it wasn't just Marla. I witnessed similar transformations in dozens of patients. I finally realized that the medical establishment's nearly exclusive focus on the biochemistry of the patient's body, often to the exclusion of the health of the patient's mind and lifestyle, was doing our patients a grave disservice.

My experience with my Marin County patients fueled the next phase of my research into what leads to optimal health and longevity. With the same passion that sent me to the library in search of proof that shifting consciousness and treating the mind can heal the body, I returned to the medical literature to search for what else, beyond the traditional health-inducing behaviors I was taught about in medical school, affects the health of the body via the health of the mind and spirit.

After researching the placebo and nocebo effects, I felt very comfortable authoritatively stating that the body is designed to repair itself and that positive belief, nurturing care, the loving consciousness of a healing presence, and the relaxation responses they induce set the stage for the body to heal itself. But are such things really enough to cure the body a decent percentage of the time? I had a sneaking suspicion it just wasn't that simple.

What about the woman who believes she will get well and finds an awesome doctor but lives with a man who cheats on her and abuses her? What about the sick person who works 12-hour days in a demeaning job that requires he sell out his integrity in order to bring home a paycheck? What about the person who smokes, drinks, eats pasta and pepperoni pizza, and lives to be 100 because his life is so full of love, vitality, and purpose that he doesn't want to leave it? I suspected there were a lot more factors involved in optimal health than we think.

Take the health nut, for example. When people are doing everything "right" when it comes to healthy behaviors—eating their organic veggies; limiting meat, dairy, gluten, and processed foods; taking supplements; exercising daily; sleeping well; avoiding addictions; seeing functional medicine doctors so they can optimize the biochemistry of the body; and so forth, we should expect them to live long, prosperous lives and die of old age while sleeping peacefully, right? So why is it that so many health nuts are sicker than others who pig out on barbecue, guzzle beer, sleep five hours a night, and veg out on the sofa in front of the boob tube?

If some health nuts are just as likely to get sick as some couch potatoes, I had to conclude that something is wrong with our definition of what constitutes a healthy lifestyle. Clearly, such healthy behaviors are a huge part of an optimally healthy life. I consider myself one of those health nuts. I drink my green juice; take my vitamins; hike, meditate, and practice yoga daily; sleep well; see a functional medicine doctor; and take measures to avoid toxins that can harm me.

And yet I have come to believe that the purely physical, biochemical realm of illness—the part you can diagnose on laboratory tests, see on radiologic studies, and explain in petri dishes under microscopes, the part that benefits from diet, exercise, avoidance of toxins, and functional medicine's positive effects on the body—is only part of the equation. It's a big part, mind you, but not the whole shebang. My experience with patients (as well as my personal experience) has led me to believe that whether patients get sick or stay healthy, whether they manage to heal or stay sick, may have even more to do with everything else that's going on in the patients' lives than with any "healthy" thing they do.

How Your Lifestyle Affects Your Body

My hypothesis—that the lifestyle choices you make can result in physiological changes in the body—extended beyond traditional healthy behaviors to include the people you interact with in your personal and professional life, how much creative freedom you experience, how spiritually connected you feel, your relationship with money, and how happy you are. People who make happy, healthy life choices, such as finding a loving, supportive life partner, having close relationships with friends and family, engaging in work they love, and treating the traumas that can lead to stress responses, tend to lead lives full of love, meaning, and fulfillment—qualities that optimize the relaxation response, counteract the stress response, and lead to better health.

We all know stress is bad for us in a vague, what-do-you-expect-me-to-do-about-it sort of way. But after my initial research, I now understood the clear link between the stress the mind experiences and the way the body breaks down. I observed how emotional stressors like loneliness, frustration at work, anger about a past trauma, money worries, spiritual disconnection, and fear could result in illness.

Had other scientists studied these kinds of links? Was there any proof to support the idea that good relationships lead to better health or that work stress leads to sickness? It was time to go back to the journals.

I set out on a mission to prove that each facet of how you live your life affects the health of your mind and, with it, the health of your body. I predicted that, in order to live a vital life, prevent disease, or optimize the chance for disease remission, you would need the following:

- Healthy relationships, including a strong network of family, friends, loved ones, and colleagues

- A healthy, meaningful way to spend your days and contribute your gifts and service to the world, whether you work outside the home or in it

- A healthy, fully expressed creative life that allows your soul to sing its song

- A healthy spiritual life, including a sense of connection to the sacred in life

- A healthy sexual life that allows you the freedom to express your authentic erotic self

- A healthy financial life, free of undue financial stress, characterized by a sense of abundance and gratitude for what you have, without greed, excessive fear of scarcity, or materialism

- A healthy, healing environment, which includes access to nature—trees, bodies of water, mountains, desert sands, gardens, or at least house plants—as well as living in a restorative sanctuary, free of toxins, natural disaster hazards, radiation, and other unhealthy factors that threaten the health of the body

- A healthy mental and emotional life, free of the heavy burdens of unhealed trauma, characterized by the ability to feel, metabolize, and move through all natural human emotions in a healthy, healing way

- A healthy lifestyle that supports the physical health of the body, such as good nutrition, regular exercise, adequate sleep, and avoidance of unhealthy toxins and addictions

Such a lifestyle may seem unrealistic, impossible even, given the unhealthy pressures, values, imbalances, and injustices of our culture. But the body is forgiving. You don't need to strive for health perfection; simple awareness that all these seemingly unrelated aspects of life have been scientifically proven to impact the health of the body can change how you view your healing journey. Each of these aspects of your life—your relationships, your work, your creative outflow, your spiritual life, your sex life, and so forth—has the power to either stress you or relax you, to be either poison or medicine. A healthy relationship elicits relaxation responses in the body. An unhealthy one flips on the stress response. A healthy spiritual life elicits healing emotions like joy, trust, connectedness, and inner peace, and the relaxation response turns on. An unhealthy spiritual life, one in which you feel judged by your spiritual community, fear punishment by a vindictive deity, or are threatened with negative outcomes like going to hell, is bound to trigger stress responses.

It's not enough to focus solely on the body without taking into account the health of the mind and its impact on your emotional life. Promoting health of the body without encouraging health of the mind is an exercise in futility. Not until we realize that our bodies are mirrors of our interpersonal, spiritual, professional, sexual, creative, financial, environmental, mental, and emotional health will we truly heal. In fact, the scientific data suggests that, at least in some instances, the health of the mind and a connection to some sort of spiritual life are equally, if not more, important to the health of the body. The body doesn't fuel how we live our lives. Instead, it is a mirror of how we live our lives. The body is a reflection of the sum of our life experiences. As psychiatrist Bessel van der Kolk, M.D., says, "The body keeps the score."

Consider the patient with pelvic pain whose pain only appears when her abusive, controlling boss walks into her office. She goes to the gynecologist, who diagnoses her with endometriosis and suggests a surgical treatment, as well as a referral to a urologist. So she visits the urologist, who puts a camera into her bladder and diagnoses her with interstitial cystitis but suggests she see a gastroenterologist, just to be certain. Then she sees a gastroenterologist, who sticks a scope up her butt and slaps her with the label of irritable bowel syndrome.

Yet nobody ever talks to her about the fact that her pain only comes when her boss is in the room. Nobody suggests that perhaps the stress of her job and her dysfunctional relationship with her boss are manifesting as physical symptoms because of repetitive stress responses in the body. Perhaps, rather than drugs or surgery, what she needs is a new job so that she can heal whatever originating traumas set her up to tolerate abuse, allowing her body to repair itself.

Sick Versus Well

If health of the body also requires health of the mental and emotional body, what shall we call this kind of health? Our health-care system doesn't even have language to describe this expanded version of health. The common definition of the word *health* doesn't take into account whether you're fulfilled at work or happy in your marriage or surrounded by a network of people who love you.

In medical school, I was taught that there are two kinds of people—sick people and well people. We all know who sick people are. They have something wrong on physical examination. They have abnormal laboratory and radiologic tests and are considered diseased or ill. They wind up taking medications, and if doctors manage to keep them from landing flat on their backs in hospitals—or even worse, dying—we breathe a sigh of relief.

If we go one step further and help them make physical lifestyle modifications that benefit the body, like diet modification or smoking cessation, and these changes cause them to feel less sick, we pat ourselves on the backs and consider our jobs well done.

Well people, on the other hand, have normal physical exams, normal laboratory and radiologic results, and are generally free of disease. If they have diseases, we've controlled them with medication, dietary changes, exercise, weight loss, or whatever is working to keep them "well."

As health-care providers, we aim to prevent well people from becoming sick people, and fortunately, greater awareness of preventive health has helped make that goal a reality. Public health education about wellness-inducing behaviors, such as good nutrition, regular exercise, smoking cessation, weight control, and cancer screening, have contributed to the wellness of the general population.

And yet, while medical technology is advancing at a rapid-fire pace and our understanding of what prevents disease continues to grow, our society is increasingly obese, hypertensive, and diabetic, suffering from heart attacks, strokes, and cancers or doped up on drugs for anxiety, depression, and bipolar disorder.

There's another category of patients who lie somewhere in between sick people and well people. They're not technically sick, but they're not exactly well either. Their blood tests come back normal. Their vital signs are stable. They're granted clean bills of health on their physicals. And yet they don't feel vital. There's an epidemic of patients like this out there.

People suffering from this epidemic come to the doctor feeling fatigued. They feel depressed and anxious. They toss and turn at night. They suffer from decreased libido. They gain weight. They numb out with a variety of addictions. And they complain of vague physical symptoms, such as muscle aches, back and neck pain, gastrointestinal disturbances, headaches, chest tightness, and dizziness.

Suspecting something is terribly wrong, patients suffering from the epidemic go to the doctor knowing something must be wrong. The doctor runs a series of tests and winds up pronouncing the patient "well." Only the patient doesn't *feel* well.

Because doctors cannot find a biochemical explanation for the symptoms these patients experience, we tend to treat them with antidepressants, pain medications, and other catchall drugs that fail to address the root cause of the issues, and the patient often fails to experience relief. So the patient goes to another doctor and starts the whole process over again because something is clearly wrong. And they're right. Something is wrong. But it's not what they think.

Many of these patients who are technically well but feel sick are suffering from the physiological consequences of repetitive stress responses that progressively break down the body. Unless the underlying stress on the nervous system is relieved, these patients often become genuinely sick. But the medical establishment doesn't seem to recognize this. Instead, they suggest that the physical symptoms are "all in your head." And they're sort of right. It starts in your head, and then it translates into the body.

The Physiology of Emotion

So how exactly does a thought or a feeling translate into physical effects all over the body? You start with a thought or a feeling—take fear, for example. A doctor tells you that you have only three months to live. Or someone injects you with something they warn you will have unpleasant side effects. Maybe you're afraid your wife is going to leave you or your boss is going to fire you or you won't be able to pay the bills or your dream won't come true or everybody will reject you because you're unlovable.

Your thoughts are powerful. Your conscious mind—which resides in the forebrain—knows you're frightened. But your lizard brain—the area near your brain stem that houses the hypothalamus—can't tell the difference between an abstract fear thought and a real live survival threat. Your lizard brain thinks you're about to die, and this stimulates the stress response, setting off the fight-or-flight mechanisms, activating the HPA axis, flipping on the sympathetic nervous system, shutting down your immune system, and getting you ready to run away from danger.

When your body is in the middle of a stress response, your body's self-maintenance and self-repair functions come to a screeching halt. These stress responses were meant to be triggered only very rarely. The healthy body is supposed to be in a relaxed state of physiological rest most of the time. If you're a caveman living in a happy tribe of people, you would only be expected to run from a cave bear once in a blue moon. The rest of the time, you'd be gathering berries, hanging around the campfire, and making little cavebabies.

Of course, our caveman ancestors didn't live very long, because of real and present dangers they faced every day, dangers we're largely protected from because of modern luxuries like ample shelter and food. But modern life has its own perils. The stressors of daily life—things like loneliness, unhappy relationships, work stress, financial stress, anxiety, and depression, all of which can stem from trauma—result in forebrain thoughts and feelings that repetitively trigger the hypothalamus to elicit stress responses. The mind knows it's just a feeling, but the lizard brain thinks you're under attack.

Feelings like fear, anxiety, anger, frustration, resentment, and other emotions associated with threat trigger the HPA axis.[1] Whether or not your body is in danger, your mind believes you are, so your hypothalamus is activated and releases corticotropin-releasing hormone (CRH) into the nervous system. CRH responds by stimulating the pituitary gland, causing it to secrete prolactin, growth hormone, and adrenocorticotropic hormone (ACTH), which stimulate the adrenal gland and cause it to release cortisol, which is in turn responsible for helping the body maintain homeostasis when the brain signals a threat.

When the hypothalamus is activated, it also turns on the sympathetic nervous system (the fight-or-flight response), causing the adrenal glands to release epinephrine and norepinephrine, which increase pulse and blood pressure and affect other physiological responses. The secretion of these hormones leads to a variety of metabolic changes all over the body.

Blood vessels traveling to the gastrointestinal tract, hands, and feet constrict, while vessels traveling to the heart, large muscle groups, and brain dilate, preferentially shunting blood to the organs that will help you escape in an emergency. Your pupils dilate so more light can get in. Metabolism speeds up in order to jolt you with a boost of energy by breaking down fat stores and liberating glucose into the bloodstream. Your respiratory rate increases and your bronchi dilate, allowing more oxygen in, and your muscles become tense and ready to sprint away from the perceived threat.

Stomach acid increases, and digestive enzymes decrease, often leading to esophageal contractions, diarrhea, or constipation. Cortisol suppresses your immune system to reduce the inflammation that would accompany any wounds the attack might inflict. Reproduction gets shut off since reproducing would take extra energy away from surviving the threat. Plus, sex and fertility are a luxury when there's danger!

Basically, your body ignores sleeping, digesting, reproducing, and self-repair and instead focuses on running, breathing, thinking, and delivering oxygen and energy in order to keep you safe. When your body is facing a physical threat, these changes help you fight or flee the threat.

As a result of the way our thoughts, beliefs, feelings, and traumas influence the autonomic nervous system, the body can't optimally relax and repair what inevitably gets ill if the stress response is stimulated and the parasympathetic nervous system shuts down by decreasing the tone of the vagus nerve. Organs get damaged. The cancer cells we naturally make every day, which usually get blasted away by the immune system, are allowed to proliferate. The effects of chronic wear and tear on the human body take their toll, and we wind up sick.

But it doesn't have to be this way. The body knows how to relax with the counterbalancing relaxation response Herbert Benson researched (see Chapter 8). When the conscious forebrain perceives safety and feels emotions like love, connection, intimacy, pleasure, and hope, the hypothalamus stops triggering the stress responses. When you feel optimistic and hopeful, loved and supported, in the flow in your professional or creative life, spiritually nourished, or sexually connected to another person, the relaxation response takes the place of the stress response. Vagal tone increases, which causes the sympathetic nervous system to shut off. Cortisol and adrenaline levels drop. The parasympathetic nervous system takes over. The immune system flips back on. And the body can go about its natural self-repair process, preventing illness and taking its stab at treating disease that already exists. When the parasympathetic nervous system is active, disease is more likely to be prevented in well people, and disease may even be treated in sick people.

While stimulation of the parasympathetic nervous system is generally supportive of healing, one exception to this may be explained by the "Polyvagal Theory" of Stephen Porges, Ph.D., which acknowledges that there are more and less primitive branches of the vagus nerve. When the more evolved branch of the vagus nerve, the myelinated branch, is stimulated, we humans respond to crises by engaging in social interactions that cause us to reach out to others who will help us heal from the stressor physically, mentally, and emotionally. But if the more primitive unmyelinated branch of the vagus nerve is stimulated, as can happen with chronic, ongoing, severe trauma, the "fight or flight" might be disabled as the "freeze" response takes over. When the more primitive unmyelinated branch of the vagus nerve takes over as stress responses become more habituated and the environment is perceived as increasingly unsafe, we tend to do the opposite of what would help us heal. We freeze, which can lead to immobilization, fainting, dissociation, and social isolation when a trauma is triggered. Instead of reaching out for the help we need, we pull away from others and collapse. This can cause us to view other humans as dangerous, which cuts us off from the love and support we need when we're in crisis. It also affects us physiologically, causing decreased heart rate variability.

Heart rate variability is a measure of general well-being and health, and the absence of it, as observed in people with frequent freeze responses, can negatively impact not only mental health issues but physical health outcomes as well, especially via the cardiovascular, respiratory, and digestive systems.[2]

Because the health of your relationships is one of the most crucial aspects of whole health, the state of your nervous system can have a huge impact on your ability to reach out to others when you're in need of healing. This is not some "woo-woo" New Age concept. It's simple physiology. We all know that love heals, but did you know that it heals not just the soul but also the body? While loneliness, anger, and resentment evoke the poisonous biochemistry of threat reactions, the desire for connection, intimacy, and a sense of belonging with family, lovers, and friends is hardwired in our DNA, and when these desires are fulfilled, our bodies respond with better health. When you find your tribe, feel loved, and surround yourself with the people who know your heart and accept you just the way you are, you optimize the body's capacity for self-repair and make your body ripe for miracles.

Components of the Cairn

In order to help my patients determine what life factors might be contributing to their health conditions, I developed a diagnostic and treatment wellness model I call the "Whole Health Cairn" based on the findings of my research, which incorporates not just how the mind can heal or harm the body, but also physical and environmental health factors that contribute to whole health. (I debuted the Whole Health Cairn in a popular TEDx talk I gave in 2011, called "The Shocking Truth about Your Health." It has now been viewed approximately 2.5 million times, which suggests to me that the mainstream is on the cusp of being ready to receive this kind of whole health medicine.)

In my medical training, I had been introduced to several wellness models—pie charts and pyramids that talked about nutrition, exercise, social health, mental health, and so forth. Most of the models included the body as the foundation upon which everything else in life builds. But something had always struck me as off about these models. Not only did I question whether the body was the foundation upon which everything else builds; I also didn't like the idea of being able to take out pieces of wellness, like you'd cut out a slice of pie. I envisioned something more intertwined, where all aspects of health were interrelated and the body was the sum total of the balance of all aspects of a wholly healthy life.

The vision for a new wellness model first came to me while I was hiking on a coastal trail near my beloved Northern California home. As an artist, I've always loved cairns—those stacks of balanced stones you see adorning beaches and marking hiking trails and sacred landmarks. I love the Zen of them, but most importantly, I love their simultaneous strength and fragility. A well-built cairn can withstand the crashing of the waves upon it, yet if you move one stone too far out of balance, the whole thing topples. All stones depend upon the others for stability.

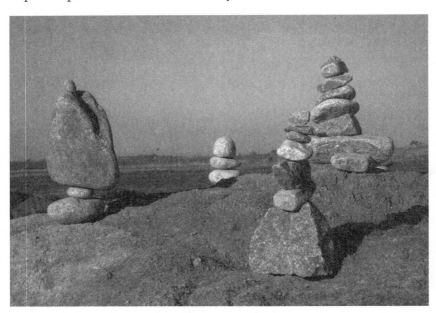

Like a cairn, the body is awe-inspiringly strong and resilient and, at the same time, fragile and easy to tip out of balance. If whole health is a stack of balanced stones, the body is the stone on top, the most precarious, the most likely to tumble if other stones shift. And as I learned on my own self-healing journey, the foundation stone, the one upon which everything else is built, is your Inner Pilot Light, that inner knowing, the healing wisdom of your body and soul that knows what's true for you and guides you, in your own unique way, back to better health.

Most wellness models teach that the body is the foundation for everything in life, that without a healthy body, everything else suffers. But we've gotten it all backward. The body isn't the foundation of your health. The body is the physical manifestation of the sum of your life experiences. When your life is out of alignment with your Inner Pilot Light and the stones of your Whole Health Cairn are out of balance, your nervous system kicks into stress response, and your body suffers. The good news is that, if you're not optimally healthy, you can cultivate shifts in your lifestyle and your consciousness that may profoundly affect your body's health.

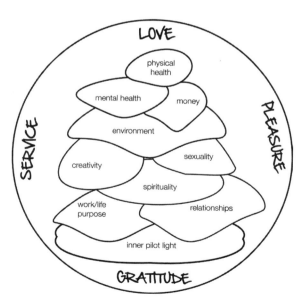

Atop the Inner Pilot Light lie all the other contributing factors that have been scientifically proven to affect health—relationships, work/life purpose, creativity, spirituality, sexuality, money, mental health, and the environment. The very top of the Whole Health Cairn is where your body's physical health rests. The Whole Health Cairn is surrounded by the "Healing Bubble" of love, gratitude, service, and pleasure—the glue I believe holds everything in balance. Love and compassion—not just from loving family, friends, and health-care providers, but especially from and for yourself—are paramount when you're embarking upon a self-healing journey. Love opens your heart, trumps fear, and paves the way for healing in all aspects of your life.

Gratitude is also important. Without gratitude, you may focus only on what's lacking in your life, rather than what you appreciate. When that happens, this process can spiral you downward into overwhelm and despair, which only increase stress responses. You have to fill your cup and appreciate what you already have before you can face the truth about what isn't working and what might need to change. Gratitude keeps you optimistic, and as we've seen, evidence shows that optimism improves your health. When you focus on gratitude, positive things flow in more readily, making you even more grateful. As long as you keep your gratitude vessel full, you'll avoid the unhealthy plunge into dark places.

Service is another part of the Healing Bubble. Dedicating our lives to serving the world connects us to one another and reminds us to focus on something bigger than ourselves. The demands of a healing journey can sometimes lead to obsessive self-absorption. Sometimes this is exactly what is needed to break co-dependent patterns of giving to the point of depletion. It's like the breath. You can't just breathe out. You must breathe in as much as you breathe out. But sometimes the healing process can lead to an unhealthy narcissism—"It's all about me and my healing journey." Finding the right balance between self-care and service can keep you inhaling and exhaling in equal measure. Tuning in to your Inner Pilot Light will help you know when to breathe in and when to breathe out. Cami Walker, author of *29 Gifts*, treated her multiple sclerosis with a practice of giving one gift per day for 29 days, which sparked an entire movement. (Join others who are doing this at 29Gifts.org.) Committing your life to serving and healing others, even in small ways, can be big-time medicine for the body, mind, and soul.

Pleasure just makes the whole darn thing more fun, while also perking up the body with health-inducing hormones such as endorphins, dopamine, nitric oxide, and oxytocin. The healing process can be hard. Dosing yourself with pleasurable, memorable experiences, laughter, sensual touch, music, art, nature, and a heaping helping of fun and play can help you ride out the rough patches. While illness, injury, or trauma can help you build up your pain tolerance, you'll need to ramp up your pleasure tolerance just as much. So don't be shy about dialing up the yum.

CHAPTER 5

LONELINESS POISONS THE BODY

How we need another soul to cling to.

— SYLVIA PLATH

When you consider how "healthy" you are, you've probably been programmed to think about your diet, your exercise regimen, your vitamins, your bad habits, your genes, and whether or not you're following doctor's orders. But have you thought about whether you feel intimately supported by a community of people you care about?

Probably not. But you should.

As it turns out, loneliness can make you sicker than smoking cigarettes, and being part of a supportive community can increase your life expectancy. Don't believe me? Let me take you back in time to Roseto, Pennsylvania, in 1961, a town where a community of Italian immigrants settled together in an enclave that recreated the Old Country in the New World.

Like its namesake in the mountains of southern Italy, Roseto Valfortore, the village of Roseto, Pennsylvania, clings to a forested ridge—this one in the Poconos, where a group of Italians who first set sail for the New World in 1882 came in search of a better life.

Because of its remoteness, few outsiders make their way into the village. But come with me into the village of Roseto, and let me show you around.

In the daytime, you'll find ghost-town-empty streets, because the children are all in school and the men and the women of Roseto are working long, tedious shifts at either the stone quarry or the blouse factory, trying to earn enough money to send their kids to college.

Two-story stone houses built along the main street of Garibaldi Avenue are clustered on the rocky hillside. Our Lady of Mount Carmel Church, which came to life when the inspiring and enterprising young priest Father Pasquale de Nisco took over, towers over the other buildings. De Nisco can be credited with much of the success of the town of Roseto. He encouraged the townspeople to plant crops, raise pigs, grow grapes, set up spiritual societies, and plan celebratory festivals. Soon thereafter, schools, shops, the blouse factory, and other evidence of culture sprang to life.

In the evening, you'll see the village of Roseto come alive as people return from work, strolling along the village's main street, stopping to gossip with the neighbors, and maybe sharing a glass of wine before heading home to change into dinner clothes. As the church bell rings, you'll see women gathering together in communal kitchens, preparing classic Italian feasts, while men push tables together in anticipation of the nightly ritual that gathers the community together over heaping piles of pasta, Italian sausage, meatballs fried in lard, and free-flowing vino.

As a community of new immigrants surrounded by English and Welsh neighbors, who turn up their noses at the Italians, the people of Roseto in 1961 are forced to look out for one another. Multigenerational homes are the norm. Everyone goes to church together. Neighbors wander in and out of one another's kitchens regularly, and holidays are joyously celebrated together. The work ethic in the community is strong. Not only does everyone work in Roseto, but they share a common mission, a life purpose that fuels their often backbreaking work. They dream of a better life for their children.

The people of Roseto take care of one another. Nobody in Roseto is left to struggle through life alone. Roseto in 1961 is living proof of the power of the clan.

This little Pennsylvania town might have gone largely unnoticed by the rest of the world had it not been brought to the attention of Dr. Stewart Wolf, a professor at the University of Oklahoma College of Medicine, who bought a summer home in the Poconos, not far away.

One summer, Dr. Wolf was asked to speak to the local medical society, and after the talk, one of the local docs invited him to go out for a drink. Over a couple of beers, the local doc mused about how strange it was that heart disease seemed far less prevalent in the little town of Roseto than in the adjoining town of Bangor.

Dr. Wolf was all ears. This conversation took place when heart attacks were happening in epidemic proportions, ringing in as the number one cause of death in men under 65. Intrigued, Dr. Wolf did his homework, scanning through death certificates from Roseto and comparing them to death certificates from the surrounding towns over a period of seven years. Amazingly, the men of Bangor had heart-attack rates paralleling the national average, but the heart-attack rate in Roseto was *half* the national average. In fact, it was nearly zero for men under 65. It wasn't just heart disease, though. The death rate from all causes was 30 to 35 percent lower than average in Roseto.

This finding merited further investigation.

As Malcolm Gladwell reports in his book *Outliers*, John Bruhn, a sociologist hired to help investigate, recalls, "There was no suicide, no alcoholism, no drug addiction, and very little crime. They didn't have anyone on welfare. Then we looked at peptic ulcers. They didn't have any of those either. These people were dying of old age. That's it."[1]

At this point Dr. Wolf and his team were committed to figuring out why the people of Roseto were so immune to disease. Attempting to answer this question, researchers poked, prodded, examined, and interviewed two-thirds of the village's adults. Dr. Wolf initially suspected they must have some Old World dietary practice making them more immune to infection. Perhaps it was all the olive oil. So he hired 11 dieticians to follow the people of Roseto into the grocery stores and watch them cook.

But that wasn't it. Unable to afford olive oil—the healthiest option—the people of Roseto cooked with lard, and they routinely ate pizza loaded with sausage, pepperoni, salami, and eggs. In fact, a shocking 41 percent of their calories came from fat.

Further, the Italian Americans in Roseto weren't physically fit. In fact, most smoked and remained sedentary, and many were obese. So what else might explain the disparity? Dr. Wolf suspected genetics. Because the Rosetans all originated from the same small village in Italy, Dr. Wolf suspected they might have inherited some disease-protective gene. So he tracked down other immigrants orig- inating from Roseto Valfortore who lived elsewhere in the United States to see if they were as healthy as their Pennsylvania cousins.

But those who originated from the same village but were scat- tered about the United States were no more healthy than average. Genetics couldn't explain it.

Dr. Wolf then evaluated Roseto's geography. Perhaps it was something in their water or the quality of the hospital where they received medical care. The same kind of evaluation went on in two neighboring towns where the rates of heart disease were in line with the national average. But it wasn't the water. They shared water with the neighboring communities of Nazareth and Bangor, where peo- ple were as sick as the general population. It wasn't the hospital, which they also shared, or the climate, which was the same.

Dr. Wolf finally realized that, if it wasn't their diet or their geog- raphy or their genes or the quality of their health care, there must be something disease-protective about Roseto itself. He concluded that a supportive, tight-knit community was a better predictor of heart health than cholesterol levels or tobacco use.

Dr. Wolf completed his initial study just as the golden age of Roseto's community life began to disintegrate. While the people of Roseto slaved away in the quarry and the blouse factory, sacrificing so their children could go to college and live the American dream, the younger generation wasn't so thrilled about life in Roseto, which to them seemed immune to modernization. When the young people went off to study at college, they brought back to Roseto new ideas, new dreams, and new people. Italian Americans started marrying non-Italians. The children strayed from the church, joined country clubs, and moved into single-family suburban houses with fences and pools.

With these changes, the multigenerational homes disbanded, and the community lifestyle shifted gears from nightly celebration to more of the typical "every man for himself" philosophy that fueled the neighboring communities. The neighbors who would regularly drop in for casual visits started phoning each other to schedule appointments. The evening rituals of adults singing songs while children played with marbles and jacks turned into nights in front of the television.

In 1971, when heart attack rates in other parts of the country were dropping because of widespread adoption of healthier diets and regular exercise programs, Roseto had its first heart attack death in someone younger than 45. Over the next decade, heart-disease rates in Roseto doubled. The incidence of high blood pressure tripled. And the number of strokes increased. Sadly, by the end of the 1970s, the number of fatal heart attacks in Roseto had increased to the national average.

As it turns out, human beings nourish one another even more than spaghetti, and the health of the body reflects this. Dr. Wolf, who continued to study the community of Roseto for many years, concluded that an isolated individual may become easily overwhelmed by the challenges of everyday life, and this kind of overwhelm can trigger stress responses in the body. An individual surrounded by a supportive community, however, relaxes. This kind of relaxation translates into positive effects on the body's physiology, leading to disease prevention and, sometimes, disease remission.

Supportive Community as Preventive Medicine

It may seem obvious to you that healthy relationships are good for the body. You might be thinking, "Duh! No news flash here."

But when's the last time your doctor asked you whether your toxic ex-husband might be causing your fibromyalgia, or your abusive mother's tongue-lashings could be predisposing you to heart disease? Have you considered whether your childhood traumas may have caused you to view others as dangerous, causing you to socially isolate and putting your body at risk?

In the rest of this chapter, I'll show how social ties and healthy relationships, including romantic relationships, healthy sexuality, and the support of a spiritual community, affect not just your happiness but also your physiology.

The reality is that loneliness causes stress, while the right kind of loving community relaxes you. The effects of stress and relaxation don't just affect the mind; they also affect the body. When you lack supportive community and feel you must handle life alone, the daily overwhelm may trigger anxiety, which the brain perceives as a threat. Such overwhelm adversely affects everything from blood pressure to kidney function. The negative consequences of overwhelm and stress can be mitigated, as it turns out, when you are nurtured by friends, relatives, and neighbors who care. In fact, this factor alone may affect your body more profoundly than what you eat, how much you drink, whether or not you smoke, or how much you exercise.[2] As I described in my TEDx talk "The #1 Public Health Issue Doctors Aren't Talking About," loneliness is an epidemic in modern societies, and those of us interested in optimizing health outcomes must address this public health risk head-on.

The Effect of Community on Life Expectancy

When you think about behaviors that will increase your life expectancy, you probably think about giving up booze, taking a daily walk, taking your vitamins, cutting back on processed foods, and wearing your seat belt more than you think about joining a club, inviting friends over for dinner, or getting a cool roommate. But perhaps it's time to rethink your preventive health strategy and start treating yourself with the medicine of positive relationships.

It's not just Roseto that shows that a supportive community impacts health. Similar studies in Peru, Israel, Borneo, and elsewhere have confirmed what researchers discovered in the small Pennsylvania village, that a community of loved ones may affect your health more than what you eat, how you exercise, and whether you have good or bad health habits.[3]

One study examining the people of Alameda County, California, found that, in every age and sex category, people with the fewest social ties were three times more likely to die over a nine-year period than those who reported the most social ties, even when you account for preexisting health conditions, socioeconomic status, smoking, alcohol consumption, obesity, race, life satisfaction, physical activity, and use of preventive health services.[4] Those with more social connections were even found to have lower rates of cancer.[5]

How much we commune with other people may prove to be as important as exercise when it comes to predicting life expectancy. A Harvard study examining the lives of almost 3,000 senior citizens found that those who gather together to go out to dinner, play cards, go on day trips, vacation with friends, go to the movies, attend sporting events, go to church, and engage in other social activities outlive their reclusive peers by an average of two and a half years. In fact, these kinds of mostly stationary social activities were found to benefit the health of the seniors as much as fitness-related activities did. The researchers concluded that social pursuits are equivalent to and independent of the merits of exercise.[6] Many more studies confirm that social ties and life expectancy are inextricably linked.[7]

The degree of social support you experience even affects the likelihood of cure if you do wind up sick. A University of California, San Francisco, study published in the *Journal of Clinical Oncology* investigated the social networks of nearly 3,000 nurses with breast cancer. This study found that the women who had been socially isolated before their breast cancer diagnosis had a 66 percent higher risk of mortality from any cause and a twofold higher risk of breast cancer mortality. The nurses who went through cancer alone were found to be four times more likely to die from their disease than those with ten or more friends supporting their journey. In fact, the data suggests that friendships may be even more health-inducing than having a spouse. In the same study, having a spouse did not show a survival benefit—but having many friendships did.[8]

The same protective effect of a strong support network was seen in a study performed at Sahlgrenska University in Sweden and published in the *European Heart Journal*, which investigated the social lives of 741 men with heart disease over a period of 15 years and determined that those with the highest measures of what they called "social integration" were the most protected against new heart attacks.[9]

In a *New Scientist* article about the effects of loneliness on health, Dr. Charles Raison, professor of psychiatry at Emory University

School of Medicine, concluded, "People who have rich social lives and warm, open relationships don't get sick and they live longer."[10]

Spiritual Community and Health

You might not consider going to church a health-inducing behavior, but it is. A study conducted by the California Public Health Foundation and published in the *American Journal of Public Health* found a strong association between attendance at religious services and lower mortality over a 28-year period for 5,286 Alameda County residents.[11] Another study, conducted at the Buck Institute for Research on Aging and also published in the *American Journal of Public Health*, evaluated religious attendance and subsequent mortality over a five-year span for 1,931 elderly residents of Marin County, California. Once again, the findings found that religious service attendance had a protective effect on life expectancy.[12]

In fact, as still another study showed, if you have heart surgery and receive support and strength from your religious community, you'll be three times more likely to be alive six months later.[13]

But why is religion so good for your health? You might think it's because people who go to church are less likely to be out boozing it up, getting high, or having one-night stands. And you'd be right. Religious people tend to behave better than their nonreligious peers.[14] In fact, many religious groups, such as Mormons or Orthodox Jews, actively promote a low-stress, positive lifestyle that advocates moderation and a harmonious family life.

But that alone doesn't explain the difference. It's more than that. People who attend religious services have larger social networks. A religious community prevents isolation and fosters better health.[15] The positive effect of spiritual community on the body's health is dramatic, possibly because places of worship encourage socialization, and people who share religious beliefs tend to take care of one another the way the people of Roseto did.

Individuals who regularly attend religious services live seven and a half years longer (almost 14 years longer for African Americans) than those who never or rarely attend religious gatherings.[16]

People who are part of a spiritual community have also been shown to have lower blood pressure and reduced risk of cardiovascular disease, lower rates of depression and suicide, lower rates of substance abuse, and stronger immune systems.[17] Mormons, whose faith leads them to gather in tight-knit communities based on shared religious beliefs, have even been shown to experience 24 percent less cancer than the general population.[18]

In the Alameda County studies, researchers found that high levels of religious involvement were associated with lower rates of circulatory diseases, digestive diseases, respiratory diseases, and just about every other disease studied. In fact, the protective effect on health of weekly attendance at a religious event was so strong that it equaled the effect of quitting smoking and exercising regularly on health.[19]

There's no question that involvement in a spiritual community prevents social isolation. Like the residents of Roseto, who took care of one another and ensured that nobody was ever lonely, religious communities often offer communal support, and the evidence suggests that the body responds with better health. But there may be other explanations for why people who participate in spiritual communities are more likely to be healthy.

In addition to the relaxation responses induced by supportive community, faith in a higher power may also induce positive emotions, which counteract stress and contribute to the state of physiological rest necessary for the body to repair itself. People with faith in a higher power are also likely to experience better health because they are better able to find meaning in the face of loss or trauma. One study showed that religious parents who lost babies to sudden infant death syndrome were better able to cope 18 months later than nonreligious parents.[20] Religious people are also more apt to forgive, which alleviates stuck emotions, such as anger and resentment, that trigger the stress response.[21]

While those who believe in a loving divinity are more likely to be happier and healthier than those who don't,[22] you don't have to subscribe to any particular religion or even believe in a higher power to reap the benefits of being more spiritual. Although traditional, institutional religious settings offer the benefit of community linked by shared belief, you can also improve your health by being more spiritually attuned through other communities, such as your local yoga studio or meditation group, ecstatic dance gatherings, or 12-step programs.

Even without community, spirituality, which has been defined by social scientists as the search for the sacred, can still offer health benefits, as you acknowledge and appreciate the sacred in life—the holiness of nature, the blessing of children, the perception of your work as a calling, the body as a vessel for love in the world, the sanctity of marriage. By imbuing the ordinary with extraordinary qualities, you open yourself up to transcendence, which can elicit relaxation in the body, leading to more happiness and, subsequently, better health. While knowing you are more than your body can induce positive health benefits, it's not all about getting out of your body and transcending this material dimension. Embodying your spirituality is also essential for optimal health. By deepening your spirituality in the body through embodiment practices, you increase somatic sensation, raise awareness of what's happening to your body, and have the potential to use the body as a compass to help you make wise, health-inducing decisions. Spiritual practices such as meditation, breath work, yoga, chant, dance, and contemplative prayer also expand your consciousness, which has its own health benefits, as often experienced by people who have had a near-death experience, a deep mystical experience in nature, a glimpse through the veils during a plant medicine journey, or as the result of meditation. When people have a mystical experience and have a chance to integrate it, they often feel less frightened and more trusting, which relaxes the nervous system and promotes better health. People who walk some sort of spiritual path are also happier, have better mental health, use fewer drugs and less alcohol, have better coping skills, and live longer than those who don't consider themselves spiritual.[23] In fact, as cancer researcher Kelly Turner, Ph.D., found in her study of people with stage 4 cancer who experienced "radical remissions," deepening one's spiritual connection is a common factor linking health outliers with seemingly miraculous recoveries.

Keep in mind that religion isn't all roses when it comes to the effect on your health. Like all facets of life, your spiritual life has the potential to stress you out as well as relax you. People for whom religion stirs up feelings of guilt, shame, repression, and fear of recrimination from a punishing God are more likely to experience repetitive stress responses, which result in poor health.[24] So it's not just spiritual life that can heal you, it's the *right* kind of spiritual life, one that is aligned with the truth of what is sacred *for you*.

Coupled Relationships and Health

If you don't think of marriage as a prescription for longevity or cohabitating with your lover as treatment for what ails you, it might be time to reconsider. While being part of a community has been demonstrated to improve health outcomes, the medical literature also suggests that being part of a coupled relationship benefits the body. The data shows that marriage affects not just your health but also your life expectancy.[25]

A University of California, Los Angeles, study that was published in the *Journal of Epidemiology and Community Health* reviewed census data and found that those who never marry are 58 percent more likely to die at a young age than those who exchange vows.[26] Happily married people also have lower blood pressure[27] and less insomnia.[28]

Are you in love but not yet married? Don't worry. It's not just married people who benefit from the health effects of being part of a couple. A New Zealand study conducted by a team at the University of Otago and published in the *British Journal of Psychiatry* examined 1,000 people and found that those in extended partnerships—regardless of whether they were married—were less likely to suffer from depression or alcohol abuse.[29]

Another study, conducted at the University of Chicago and Northwestern University and published in the journal *Stress*, investigated 500 M.B.A. students—almost half of whom were married or in relationships. The students were instructed to play a series of economic computer games, which they believed were part of their exams. Saliva samples were taken before and after to measure levels of hormones, such as the stress hormone cortisol. To create an environment of stress, each student was told that the test was a course requirement and that it would impact his or her future career placement.

Concentrations of stress hormones increased in all participants, but unpaired individuals of both sexes had higher levels of stress hormones than those who were in committed relationships. Researchers concluded: "Although marriage can be pretty stressful, it should make it easier for people to handle other stressors in their lives."[30]

While some people are happy to stay single, most people yearn for intimate connection with a romantic partner. We are biologically programmed to mate, and the positive benefits on health demonstrated by those in happily coupled relationships suggest a survival advantage in such mating that benefits the body. How do coupled relationships improve health? Most likely through the impact on your emotional health. When you feel loved, supported, and nurtured in a relationship, when you have help navigating the daily details of life, when you don't feel like you have to tackle all of life's inevitable challenges solo, your nervous system experiences fewer stress responses and elicits more relaxation responses, and the physiology of the body responds accordingly.

Keep in mind that merely pairing off isn't the answer. Coupled relationships can be the source of both stress and relaxation. It's not just any relationship that will benefit your health—it's the right one. When it comes to your health, you're actually better off single than in a bad relationship.[31] An unhappy marriage can harm your health, as demonstrated by an Ohio State University study published in the journal *Cancer*, which examined 100 patients with breast cancer and demonstrated that those in bad marriages fared less well than those in happy marriages.[32]

Abusive marriages also pose health risks, not just relating to injury, but because of other causes of illness that likely result from the chronic repetitive stress responses induced by the repetitive trauma of abuse, which often retriggers early childhood traumas. Married or cohabitating women who are victims of domestic abuse are more likely to get sick.[33] So don't stay in a bad relationship just because you think it will benefit your health. Remember, relationships can be medicine or poison. The key is to foster relationships that initiate relaxation responses rather than those that trigger stress responses.

Have you lost a partner? When one half of a couple dies, it's especially important for the surviving partner to seek support from others. One study showed that men and women who had lost a spouse from sudden, accidental death were much more likely to get sick themselves. However, if the widows and widowers confided in others close to them, they had fewer health problems and were more likely to be happy.[34]

Sexuality and Health

Another well-documented health advantage people in coupled relationships usually enjoy is sex. With all the warnings about the dangers of sex—sexually transmitted diseases, rape, sexual abuse, and the risks of pregnancy—you might not realize that sex can be good for your health. But studies show that the benefits of a healthy sexual relationship with an intimate partner improve the health of the body in remarkable ways.

Those with healthy sexual lives live longer, have a lower risk of heart disease and stroke, get less breast cancer, bolster their immune systems, sleep better, appear more youthful, enjoy improved fitness, have enhanced fertility, get relief from chronic pain, experience fewer migraines, suffer from less depression, and enjoy an improved quality of life.[35]

The evidence is mounting. Sex isn't just fun—it's good for your health! While some of the benefits of an active sex life may be attributable to the physical workout of a good romp in the hay, the positive effects of a healthy sex life on the mind—eliciting the physiological relaxation response and its counteracting effects on the stress response—may even more dramatically affect the physiology of the body.

But like all facets of how we live our lives, sex has the potential to stress you out too. If you have unhealed sexual trauma, as so many people do, this poses a significant risk to your physical health, but the good news is that it can be treated. A meta-analysis of the long-term physical health sequelae of childhood sexual abuse showed higher rates of many subsequent physical health symptoms, including gastrointestinal and gynecologic symptoms, chronic pain, cardiopulmonary symptoms, obesity, and impaired general health.[36]

It's not just sexual trauma that can put you at risk of physical disease. If you're sexually frustrated, feeling distrustful of your partner, cheating on your spouse, losing your libido, or experiencing pain with sex, your sex life can also trigger stress responses. The key to using your sex life as a tool for preventive health and disease treatment is to ensure that it's healthy and leaves you feeling relaxed, not stressed. If your sex life is stressing you out, addressing the underlying issues coming between you and a healthy sex life is crucial. Well-trained sex counselors or trauma therapists with expertise in sexual trauma can make all the difference.

The Physiology of Loneliness

So what is it about living in a close-knit community, gathering together with others who share your faith, being part of a coupled relationship, having lots of friends, and enjoying sexual intimacy with another person that stimulates better health?

Healthy relationships are medicine for the mental and emotional body, and as we've already seen, the mind has powerful effects on the physiology of the body. So many people, especially those in the developed world, suffer from social isolation. While social isolation can sometimes be positive—a way to recharge the mind through retreats, meditation, personal time, and other nourishing, health-inducing activities—chronic social isolation can lead to loneliness, and multiple studies demonstrate that loneliness can trigger stress responses in the body, the same kind of fight-or-flight responses fear of bodily harm can elicit. Conversely, unhealed trauma can elicit the freeze response that leads to social isolation, which can cause a vicious cycle that interferes with healing. The good news is that this can be reversed. Some might need professional help to treat the underlying traumas that lead to social isolation and loneliness, but sometimes all it takes is the decision to make a change.

Everyone feels lonely from time to time, but for some people loneliness becomes the norm. Canadian psychologist Vello Sermat, who studies loneliness, estimates that 10 to 30 percent of people suffer from a pervasive feeling of loneliness.[37] In another study, 16 percent of people responding to a newspaper advertisement described themselves as being "lonely most or all of the time."[38] Among lonely people, 37 percent describe their health as "poor" or "very poor."[39]

As Robert Putnam put it in *Bowling Alone*, "As a rough rule of thumb, if you belong to no groups but decide to join one, you cut your risk of dying over the next year in half. If you smoke and belong to no groups, it's a toss-up statistically whether you should stop smoking or start joining. These findings are in some way heartening. It's easier to join a group than to lose weight, exercise regularly, or quit smoking."[40]

As it turns out, psychologist John Cacioppo, who has devoted his life's work to studying the effects of social isolation and loneliness on the body, agrees that curing loneliness is as good for your health as giving up smoking. According to Cacioppo, lonely people are physiologically different from people with strong social networks when it comes to cortisol-signaling genes, the inflammatory response, and the immune system.[41] Lonely people demonstrate higher diastolic blood pressure responses to stress, altered immune response, and greater cortisol responses to stress.[42]

Lonely people have also been shown to have higher rates of heart disease, breast cancer, Alzheimer's disease, and suicidal thoughts.[43] Loneliness even affects mortality rates after coronary artery bypass surgery. A Swedish study examining 1,290 patients undergoing heart surgery found that patients who agreed with the statement "I feel lonely" had significantly higher mortality rates postoperatively.[44]

In studies comparing lonely and non-lonely individuals, lonely people were found to have significantly altered cardiovascular function, including higher levels of peripheral resistance in the blood vessels, higher blood pressure, lower levels of blood vessel–relaxing carbon monoxide, and alterations in heart rate and cardiac contractility that mimic what happens when the body is facing a threat.

Researchers also suspect that lonely individuals suffer from poor-quality sleep, and limited sleep is known to lower glucose tolerance, elevate cortisol levels, and increase fight-or-flight sympathetic nervous system activation. These effects mirror what is seen in normal aging and may explain why the body suffers in lonely individuals.[45]

Chronically lonely individuals have been found to have higher salivary cortisol levels across the course of a day, suggesting more discharges of corticotropin-releasing hormone and activation of the HPA axis, which triggers stress responses.[46] Multiple studies also demonstrate that loneliness leads to suppressed immune function, which can alter the body's ability to fight infection, mount an attack against cancer cells, and repair itself internally.[47]

Cacioppo suggests that ending loneliness is not so much about spending more time with people; he thinks it is all about altering our *attitude* toward others. Traumatized individuals may come to view other human beings as potentially dangerous. My introverted housemate, who experienced a lot of childhood trauma, has a T-shirt emblazoned with the words "Ew, People," which always makes me laugh. Because of my own traumas, I can relate to that feeling, and I imagine some of you can too. When we don't know how to protect ourselves around others, when our boundaries are not shored up and protected, when we feel we are in danger when we're around others, harmful stress hormones and other fear chemicals are triggered. Such intense feelings can make us isolate, and this can lead to loneliness. When we heal the loneliness, the body may follow.

The mind might recognize loneliness for what it is—a feeling of disconnection, of not belonging, of feeling unloved—but the lizard brain only knows one way to communicate with the rest of the body: "Houston, we have a problem!" While the mind might be able to differentiate between facing up against a wild animal on the prowl and feeling lonely, the slew of hormones the mind spews out in response to a threat is exactly the same in the body. When the mind signals the alert, your hypothalamus, pituitary gland, and adrenal glands come to life, and a surge of stress hormones, such as adrenaline, norepinephrine, and cortisol, course through your bloodstream, galloping off like Paul Revere to tell all the other organs there's a wild animal on the loose.

Normally, when the lizard brain perceives that the lion is gone, the stress-response systems reset, alerting the organs to go back to business as usual. But if you feel chronically lonely, your body may switch on the stress-response alert and leave it on, which, in time, can activate the unmyelinated branch of the vagus nerve and lead to social isolation. The depleted stress hormones can lead to a freeze response, which can not only damage your health but also shorten your life. When loneliness is known to pose as much health risk as smoking, shouldn't doctors be prescribing social support, trauma treatment, and alleviation of loneliness as part of an optimally healthy lifestyle?

All Relationships Are Not Created Equal

The scientific data supports the notion that healthy relationships affect your nervous system, which in turn affects the body. But, clearly, all relationships are not created equal. Many lonely individuals have chosen to be alone as a response to traumatic relationships that can harm the mind and the body. We know that childhood abuse or neglect can shorten a person's lifespan.[48] People who endure relationships characterized by conflict or hostility suffer physically and emotionally.[49] Clearly, physically abusive marriages can injure or kill you. When your clan is a street gang that engages in regular shoot-outs, your health is obviously at risk. When your community revolves around injecting heroin together, your health would be better served by being alone.

While these examples of how the wrong relationships can harm you may seem obvious, you might be less aware of how other, more subtle types of unsupportive social ties may damage your health. You may not realize that when your church community judges you because you don't conform to social norms, your mind is likely to mount a stress response that could negatively affect your body. When your family routinely chews you a new one every time you go home to visit, Sunday afternoon family dinners might not be as beneficial to your health as they were in Roseto. When you're hanging out with the mommy crowd from your kid's school, but you're feeling like it's unsafe to be authentic, your body may sense a threat.

It's old news that unhealthy relationships are bad for you. This is no shocker. You probably have relationships in your life you know are harming you, but you may not realize how they affect the physiology of the body. When you get cancer, you may not automatically leap to the conclusion that your emotionally abusive marriage could have weakened your immune system through chronic activation of the stress response or that your immune system may have shut down because you were constantly caregiving others and neglecting your own needs. When you have a heart attack, you may not link it to your sister, who verbally beats you up every time you call, or your "friend," who cuts you down every time you see each other and gossips about you behind your back. When you're struggling with chronic pain, you may not realize that your physical symptoms may be the result of your co-dependent relationship with your son. As Gabor Maté, M.D., author of *When the Body Says No*, teaches, when you can't protect your own boundaries and say no when you mean it, your body may say no for you.

Although the data suggests that we need the company of other humans in order to be optimally healthy, what we really need are healthy, genuine relationships that allow us to be who we really are without judgment or criticism. Social contact simply isn't enough. If you surround yourself with people who make you feel like it isn't safe to be vulnerable, your body will manifest a stress response.

Other negative relationship dynamics, such as aggression, hate, or withdrawal of love, stimulate the stress response, whereas love, nurturing, compassion, and feelings of attachment and belonging trigger the release of hormones, such as oxytocin, dopamine, and endorphins, that induce relaxation and feelings of pleasure.

In other words, be social. Avoid loneliness. Surround yourself with friends and family. But be mindful of the relationships you choose to bring into your life. Choose your inner circle wisely, and make sure, at the end of the day, you feel supported by those in your social community, rather than judged, criticized, bullied, pressured, or threatened.

As a general rule, human beings are social animals. Historically, bonding in community offered an evolutionary advantage in a world rife with threats. Deep in our souls, we long for love, belonging, and human connection. Yes, some of us are introverts and some are extroverts, so as a fellow introvert, I'm not suggesting you need to force yourself to be a social butterfly. In her book *Quiet: The Power of Introverts in a World That Can't Stop Talking*, Susan Cain makes the case that it can be traumatizing for people inclined toward introversion to be pressured to be extroverted. Introverts need time alone to recharge, regulate their nervous systems, and heal.

That said, don't confuse unhealed trauma or poor boundaries for introversion. Some of us have had our hearts broken and seek isolation as a protective mechanism against further trauma to the heart. Some don't know how to protect ourselves unless we're alone. Some have a greater need for human connection, while others find that what our minds and bodies need in order to elicit physiological relaxation are hours of solitary meditation. Ultimately, you must tap into the healing wisdom of your own intuition in order to determine what will nourish you, your mind, and your body.

It's hard to open yourself up to relationships when you feel unsafe. Opening your heart and exposing your soft underbelly feels like the last thing you want to do when your heart has been traumatized, as so many of ours have. But it's essential to get help, treat your traumas, and learn to set and enforce healthy boundaries so you can open up around others. Shame, secrecy, and isolation are the enemies of the healing process.

The Power of Vulnerability

As a professor at the University of Houston, Brené Brown, author of *Daring Greatly, Rising Strong,* and *The Gifts of Imperfection,* among others, studies shame, fear, and the power of vulnerability to transform shame into intimate connection with other human beings. In the viral TEDx talk "The Power of Vulnerability," as well as in her books, Brown discusses the role of shame and how it leads to social isolation. She teaches that the courage to be vulnerable, the cultivation of compassion for the imperfections of others, and the creation of healthy boundaries set the stage for healthy relationships.

In *The Gifts of Imperfection*, Brown writes, "If we want to live and love with our whole hearts, and if we want to engage with the world from a place of worthiness, we have to talk about the things that get in the way—especially shame, fear, and vulnerability." She describes shame as the fear of being unlovable and states that it exists for us all: "To feel shame is to be human."

How we shame ourselves and what we shame ourselves about varies from individual to individual but runs the gamut—body image, work, money, relationships, addictions, parenting, sex, aging, family, and more. But there's good news. If we're all capable of feeling shame, we're all also capable of what Brown calls "shame resilience"—the ability to recognize shame when it rears its ugly head, move through it in a healthy way, hang on to our sense of worthiness and authenticity, and use it to develop more courage, compassion for others who feel their own shame, and connection with others as a result.

According to Brown, the difference between guilt and shame is that guilt implies "I did something bad," while shame suggests "I am bad." While guilt is often a motivator to live with more integrity, shame makes us want to be swallowed up by the earth. When you're in the swirl of a shame attack, the feeling is so intolerable that you may avoid relationships just to avoid feeling shame. But Brown recommends, instead of isolating and trying to protect ourselves with inauthentic masks, discerning who can be trusted and then mustering up the courage to be vulnerable and authentic, embracing self-compassion, letting go of perfectionism, and cultivating what she calls "Wholeheartedness," the practice of living and loving with a whole heart.

In her research on shame, fear, and vulnerability, Brown found that Wholehearted people live lives full of worthiness, rest, play, trust, faith, intuition, hope, authenticity, love, belonging, joy, gratitude, and creativity, while avoiding perfectionism, numbing, certainty, exhaustion, self-sufficiency, being cool, fitting in, judgment, and scarcity.[50]

Every day is an opportunity to deepen your connections to the people you value. When you let your heart feel, become resilient to shame, end your judgments of others, learn the art of forgiveness, practice being authentic, and lay bare your soul, you allow your mind to work its wonders, optimizing the body for its natural state of self-repair.

Rx for Loneliness

If you live a solitary life and have either given up trying to be more social or chosen to remain alone, you may be able to counter-balance some of the negative effects on health caused by loneliness and social isolation. In Chapter 8, I'll be teaching you some techniques you can employ at home to elicit relaxation responses and tone down stress responses.

If you're lonely and motivated to improve your health, or if you're involved in toxic relationships and need an antidote to the harm these relationships may be inflicting on your body, stay tuned. In Chapter 9, you'll have the chance to diagnose any relationship imbalances in your life and come up with an action plan for how you might relieve loneliness and enjoy the health benefits of healthy relationships.

Until then, I want you to know that the best way to alleviate loneliness is to tap into the essential nature of who you really are. Let the world see your real, authentic, beautiful fabulousness. So many of us expend so much energy trying to be someone we're not in order to fit in. In our efforts to be accepted, we lose a part of ourselves, and our health suffers as a consequence.

The truth is that people aiming to be socially acceptable are trying to hit the bull's-eye of a constantly moving target of acceptability, which means staying on top of trends, comparing themselves to others, sacrificing what they really love for what they think others love, and adhering to artificial standards of conformity. The cooler you try to be, the more isolated you'll feel. As Brené Brown says, "The number one barrier to belonging is fitting in." It's a guaranteed recipe for loneliness. It's also a heavy price to pay, one that can leave you not only lonely but also sick.

You may be tempted to seek social acceptance so you won't feel like a misfit or wind up hurt. We all want to feel loved and accepted. We long to belong. But at what price? Is it worth selling out who you are and replacing the real you with some plastic version constantly re-created to fit today's elusive acceptability factor (which you can guarantee is different than yesterday's)?

Nope.

Stripping off your masks and letting your inner radiance shine forth might not be "cool," but it allows an opportunity for deep connection. It takes real courage to be unapologetically uncool—and there's really nothing cooler in my book than people brave enough to be who they really are, even when it flies in the face of everything popular culture commands you to be. When you're brave enough to be unapologetically *you*, and you've treated enough of your traumas to allow yourself to be truly seen, in all of your glorious radiance and your darkest shadows, you become a magnet for all the others who long to be fearless enough to do the same. That, my friend, is a surefire way to alleviate loneliness.

CHAPTER 6

DEATH BY OVERWORK

Unnatural work produces too much stress.

— BHAGAVAD GITA

You already know that workplace hazards can harm your health. The soldier dies in battle. The policeman gets caught in the criminal's crosshairs. A construction worker falls from a 20-story building. A researcher experiences a biohazard accident and winds up with a rare infectious disease.

What you do during your workday can clearly affect the body. But it affects the body not just through physical hazards. It also affects the body through the power of your thoughts and emotions, which respond to what you do during your workday by either triggering stress responses or initiating relaxation responses. You know work has the potential to stress you out. But you may also have experienced times at work when you're doing what you love, you're in the flow, you feel a sense of mission and purpose, and you're grateful to be doing something that matters. Such feelings can benefit the body as much as stress responses harm it.

We all know that work stress is poisonous and can translate into physical symptoms. Anyone who has ever gotten a migraine after a deal went bad or stiff shoulders after the boss criticized him can attest to that.

But has your doctor ever prescribed doing work you love as treatment for your tumor or suggested that quitting your job might cure your irritable bowel syndrome? When was the last time you diagnosed your job stress as the root cause of your stroke or credited your professional fulfillment with the spontaneous remission of your chronic disease?

Perhaps it's time for a paradigm shift.

You may not have thought much about how your work affects your health. If you're sick, you may have assumed that your illness is the result of a defective gene, poor diet, insufficient exercise, a biochemical imbalance, or plain old bad luck—and this may indeed be true. But work stress may be a contributing, even causative, factor. You might be surprised to realize that the prescription for your illness might not be a pill or surgery. It might be finding new ways to handle work stress, making changes in your current job in order to reduce anxiety, or even finding a new career.

As it turns out, you really can work yourself to death. You can also follow your bliss back to health. In Japan, there is more awareness about the effect of job stress on health. They even have a word for it: *karoshi*, which is defined as "death by overwork."

Like many of the other 7.7 million Japanese who slog their way through 60-plus-hour work weeks, Satoru Hiraoka was a good soldier, the kind who prioritized the company first and his family last while banishing any frivolous notions like leisure time, weekends off, or vacation days. For over 28 years, Hiraoka, a middle manager at the Tsubakimoto Seiko precision bearing factory in Osaka, dutifully worked 12- to 16-hour days, often capping out at 95 hours of work each week.

This was no exaggeration. Review of Hiraoka's time cards showed that in the year prior to his untimely death, Hiraoka put in over 1,400 hours of overtime. Like the perfect employee, he never called in sick, never took a hangover day, and never skipped out on work to catch his child's school play. He was the ideal *kigyo-senchi* ("corporation soldier").[1]

Then one day, on February 23, 1988, after putting in a 15-hour day, the 48-year-old came home from work and suffered what the doctors called "sudden cardiac insufficiency." He died instantly.

Hiraoka's death, and tens of thousands of others just like his, might have gone unnoticed had a group of Japanese occupational medicine specialists and cardiologists not been studying the phenomenon. These doctors noticed that people who were overworked were at increased risk of dying of unexpected cardiovascular and cerebral diseases, such as heart attack and stroke.

The first case had been reported in 1969, when a worker died of a stroke at the age of 29.[2]

But it wasn't until 1987 that the Japanese ministry of labor began collecting statistics on karoshi. Japanese officials estimate that since that time, approximately 10,000 cases of karoshi have occurred each year.[3] Some lawyers and scholars claim that the number of karoshi deaths in Japan equals or exceeds the number of traffic-accident fatalities each year.[4]

According to Shunichiro Tajiri, head of the Osaka-based Social Medical Study Institute, karoshi victims are typically otherwise healthy men in their 40s and 50s who are middle managers in stressful jobs that require them to work more than 12-hour days six or seven times a week. Just before dying, most complain of varying combinations of dizziness, nausea, severe headache, and stomachache. In 95 percent of karoshi cases, death occurs within 24 hours of the onset of severe symptoms, though milder symptoms sometimes precede the severe ones.

In a *Chicago Tribune* article, Tajiri said, "In each case, the men were healthy, with no evidence of any disease. They simply worked themselves to death."

Hiraoka's widow is one of many Japanese who filed karoshi claims to receive workers' compensation benefits. But because karoshi is itself not quite a disease—it's a constellation of what are believed to be stress-induced physiological changes—and because it's often hard to prove that a victim's death is directly related to too much work stress or long hours, these benefits can be tougher to secure than those given to people who die from on-the-job accidents.[5] Nonetheless, karoshi claims are rising, and workers' compensation benefit payouts are too.

Death by Overwork in the United States

It's not just the Japanese who are working themselves to death, and it's not a new phenomenon. In June of 1863, a London newspaper reported a story, entitled "Death from Simple Over-work," about a 20-year-old woman who died after working days that averaged over 16 hours a day (up to 30-hour shifts during the busy season) in a garment factory. While this might sound like the stuff of Dickensian novels, the truth is that it's happening right now in the United States, as much as it is in Japan or England.

The Information Age has transformed us into workaholics who no longer have the forced respite of snail mail and hand-delivered memos. Now it's not just doctors who are on call 24/7. It's most of us. The advent of e-mail, cell phones, pagers, fax machines, laptops, and iPads means we are accessible almost all the time, and increasingly poor employee health is reflecting it. Not that poor health stops employees from coming in to work. A study conducted by the health insurer Oxford Health Plans found that one in five Americans come to work even if they're ill, injured, or seeing a doctor that day.[6] The same sort of work obsession has about a third of employed Americans failing to use accrued vacation time, according to a survey by Expedia.com.

Similarly, about a quarter of British workers do not take all their vacation time, and in France, many don't either. The difference is that most Europeans get much more vacation time—an average of 26 days for the British and 37 for the French—compared with 14 days for the average American. Another difference is that, while 137 countries mandate paid vacation time, the United States is the only industrialized country that does not.[7]

This failure to take a break has actually been associated with early death. One study, published in *Psychosomatic Medicine* in 2000, looked at 12,000 men over nine years and found that those who failed to take annual vacations had a 21 percent higher risk of death from all causes and were 32 percent more likely to die of a heart attack.[8]

In another study, published in the *American Journal of Epidemiology*, researchers at Johns Hopkins evaluated data collected from patients in the Framingham Heart Study over a period of 20 years and found that women who vacationed once every 6 years or less often were almost eight times more likely to develop coronary heart disease or have a heart attack than women who vacationed twice a year.[9]

There's a good reason why Workaholics Anonymous is now an active 12-step program in the United States as well as in many other countries. Although most of the data on karoshi comes from Japan, the International Labour Organization released statistics showing that the United States far exceeds Japan when it comes to overwork. Our doctors and our government have yet to recognize karoshi as a distinct disease or award workers' compensation benefits the way the Japanese do, and because we don't track it, it's hard to say how frequently work stress manifests as death in the United States. But you can bet it affects the health of many.

Types of Job Stress

People who experience stress at work get their stress responses repetitively triggered throughout the workday. Imagine the red-faced, pot-bellied prosecuting attorney screaming at the quivering, weepy witness—like a cartoon character with steam coming out of his ears—until the attorney keels over in the middle of the court-room with a heart attack. Then there's the type-A Wall Street stock trader who spends 16 hours a day screaming bloody murder until her blood pressure skyrockets and she has a stroke at the age of 42. Keep in mind that the meek, mild-mannered people who work for those blustery bosses are firing stress responses in their bodies too as the result of subtle or not-so-subtle abuse.

Golden handcuffs are alive and well, and many high-powered professionals are coming in at dawn and staying until bedtime, working 100-hour weeks in exchange for big, fat paychecks. Other, less privileged workers slave away just as hard, minus the fancy pay-out. Exceptionally long hours and unusually demanding workloads face physicians, investment bankers, business consultants, truckers, pilots, attorneys, and countless others.

Job stressors vary, but the stress affects the body in similar ways. There's the stress caused by interpersonal conflict, which may be experienced by lawyers, debt collectors, customer service repre-sentatives, or anyone who is bullied by co-workers, supervisors, or customers. There's the stress experienced by people in high-stakes careers, such as doctors, nurses, firefighters, soldiers, air traffic controllers, commercial airline pilots, and criminal attorneys, where one wrong move can ruin someone's life—or end it.

There's the stress of jobs that expect you to sell your soul or sacrifice your integrity, like the advertising executive expected to spearhead a campaign for an unhealthy product, the white-collar insider commanded to keep quiet about fraudulent activities the company might be engaging in, the soldier ordered to carry out an operation he doesn't believe is ethical, and the politician who sacrifices her own values in order to get a law passed.

There's also the stress of feeling powerless or lacking control in the workplace, which might be experienced by the nurse who knows the doctor has ordered the wrong treatment but must follow orders anyway or by the person low on the corporate ladder who has big ideas but doesn't think his little voice matters.

Other types of work stress fall under the heading of organizational constraints—tedious, frustrating hurdles that get in the way of getting the job done well, such as meddling co-workers, limited access to necessary information, or lacking the authority to do what needs to be done in order to successfully complete a task.

There's the stress of role confusion, which comes about when you don't understand what is expected of you or whether you're meeting expectations. There's also the stress of conflicting messages, when different members of a work environment deliver countering instructions that leave you scratching your head.

While the mind interprets all these stressors as different, the lizard brain perceives the same thing in each case—*threat*. The physiological stress response flips on. Regardless of what causes the stress, the body manifests a physiological response similar to what happens when a person suffers from chronic loneliness. Because the mind communicates with the body via hormones, the physiological response is the same whether you're listening to your boss rant at you, trying to calm down an angry client, or putting out a fire in a burning building.

So next time you choose to work overtime, your boss screams at you, or you're put in a work situation that leaves you feeling powerless, keep in mind that you might be taking years off your life by taxing your heart, wearing out your blood vessels, irritating your digestive tract, exhausting your adrenal glands, weakening your immune system, and stressing your pancreas.

Is it really worth it? It's easy to rationalize enduring stressful situations when you're working your way up the corporate ladder, struggling to keep your job in a lagging economy, or worrying about how you'll pay the rent if you don't make those sales. But are you really willing to withdraw years from your life account to make more money, attract more clients, or impress your boss?

Consider, instead, making an investment in your health for years to come by setting boundaries and implementing self-care at work. In Chapter 8, we'll talk about ways to protect your body from job stress, and in Part III of the book, we'll discuss how to ensure that your work is aligned with your highest truth in order to optimize your health. Until we get there, suffice it to say that work stress is not benign. In order to live a vital, long life, it's important to find ways to feel peaceful and relaxed at work.

Typical Symptoms of Work Stress

When exposed to stress at work, the body whispers before it begins to yell. Before you collapse of a heart attack, keel over from a stroke, or wind up with cancer, you're likely to experience milder physical symptoms, such as backache, headache, eye strain, insomnia, fatigue, dizziness, appetite disturbances, and gastrointestinal distress.

Consider the following symptoms warning signs of more serious diseases in the making.

Backaches

Several studies have shown that backaches, such as those related to arthritis and fibromyalgia, increase in response to daily stressors such as work.[10] The relationship between work stress and backaches (as well as other types of musculoskeletal pain) is believed to occur because repetitive stress and activation of the HPA axis depletes cortisol and raises prolactin levels, thereby increasing the body's sensitivity to pain by suppressing the immune system and increasing inflammation.[11]

Headaches

As anyone who has ever pulled an all-nighter and suffered a migraine can attest, work stress can also cause headaches, most likely because pain-signaling pathways in the brain become hypersensitized in times of stress. Once the brain is overly sensitized to painful stimuli, even the slightest twinge may excite nerves in the brain, causing pain and muscle tension.[12]

Eye Strain

Occupational stress can also lead to eye strain, which includes itchy, heavy, or sore eyes as well as blurred or double vision, believed to be caused by inflammation and increased responsiveness to pain stimuli in and around the eyes. Certain workplace tasks, such as computer use, can also increase eye muscle fatigue.[13]

Insomnia

Notorious for keeping us up at night, work stress accounts for more lost sleep than any other cause.[14] A Swedish study showed that 10 to 40 percent of the working-age population reported work-related insomnia.[15] Scientists theorize that higher levels of ACTH and cortisol triggered by the stress response reduce surges of night-time melatonin levels, which we need for restful sleep.[16]

Fatigue

Obviously, if your job is affecting your sleep, you're likely to feel fatigued, but other physiological factors may also make you feel fatigued when you're stressed at work, even if you're sleeping well. Although its mechanism is poorly understood, fatigue is one of the most common symptoms people experience when they're stressed by work. Work stress also increases the risk of chronic fatigue syndrome.[17] Theories link work-related fatigue to depleted cortisol levels, as well as to a genetic predisposition to stress-mediated fatigue.[18] What is clear is that individuals respond to the chemical alterations caused by stress in unique ways, so some people are more likely than others to feel fatigue when they experience work stress.[19]

Dizziness

As if some jobs aren't dizzying enough, workplace stress makes some people experience dizziness, believed to be related to changes in heart rate, blood pressure, and respiratory rate caused by stimulation of the sympathetic nervous system.[20] Alterations in these vital signs, particularly elevations in respiratory rate, can lead to hyperventilation, which alters the acid-base balance of the body, disrupting the nervous system's responses to balance and coordination via the cerebellum and the eighth cranial nerve.[21]

Appetite Disturbances

Depending on your unique physiology, work stress can either increase or decrease appetite, leading to weight loss or weight gain, although the most common response to work stress is decreased appetite.[22] In one study, 21 percent of respondents reported a significant loss of appetite following a stressful event.[23] Emotional stressors can trigger the brain to release ACTH and melanocyte-stimulating hormone (MSH), which can lead to loss of appetite and subsequent weight loss.[24]

Paradoxically, stimulation of the sympathetic nervous system may also cause the stomach to release the amino acid ghrelin, which makes you feel hungry and can lead to weight gain.[25] While these mechanisms come into play at the time of stress initiation, chronic work stress also affects appetite via stress-induced cortisol production. When cortisol levels are high, body fat tends to increase, and when cortisol levels are exhausted, release of the signaling peptide leptin decreases appetite.

Gastrointestinal Distress

Work stress commonly leads to gastrointestinal disorders such as nausea, heartburn, abdominal cramps, diarrhea, and irritable bowel syndrome, most likely mediated by the increased amounts of ACTH generated during the stress response. In response to ACTH, gastric emptying is delayed, which can lead to stomachaches and abdominal cramping. Heartburn can worsen, not only because stomach acid levels increase, but also because the stress response reduces the stomach's pain threshold, increasing the perception of pain in response to heartburn and predisposition to stomach ulcers.[26] The stress response also lowers the stomach's ability to expand, which stimulates contractions of muscles in the colon and can lead to diarrhea and other symptoms of irritable bowel syndrome, most likely related to overproduction of CRH.[27]

Work Stress and Life-Threatening Disease

While backaches, stomachaches, and insomnia might not strike you as serious health issues, they are early warning signs, resulting from the body's stress response. These symptoms may be similar to the symptoms lonely people experience. The average American experiences 50 brief stress-response episodes each day, and lonely people or those unduly stressed about work experience even more, requiring the body to devote energy to maintaining healthy homeostasis.

At first, the body keeps up. But over time, the body gets tired, and things go wrong. Frequent elevations in blood pressure result in thickening and tearing of blood vessel walls. Excessive production of fatty acids and glucose causes plaques that lead to heart disease. Chronic muscle tension and inflammation leads to pain and musculoskeletal disorders. Overproduction of cortisol suppresses the immune system, predisposing the body to infection and cancer.[28]

Chronic stimulation of the stress response caused by job stress can lead to heart disease, thyroid disease, ulcers, autoimmune disease, obesity, diabetes, sexual dysfunction, depression, anorexia nervosa, Cushing's syndrome, chronic fatigue syndrome, inflammatory disease, and cancer.[29] One study even showed that those in a hostile work environment are more likely to die young.[30] Another study of 7,000 people demonstrated that, while being employed is generally better for your health than being unemployed, it's better to be unemployed than employed in a badly paid, demanding, unsupportive job where you have little power or control.[31]

So while you might enjoy the paycheck a stressful job delivers, keep in mind that you may be paying a price even greater than what they're paying you.

Financial Stress and Health

If you're in a stressful job and suspect your health is suffering as a consequence, you may think about cutting back your hours, quitting your job, or switching careers. But if you're one of those people, the boogeyman in your lizard brain is probably whispering evil nothings like "You can't afford to quit, you moron. How will you ever pay the bills?"

This is a very real concern for many people. Your body might decompensate when you're in a stressful work environment, but the fear of job loss can amplify these feelings further.

Usually, work stress and financial stress are linked. It's a catch-22, really, because financial stress can be just as harmful to your health as work stress or loneliness. Studies linking wealth and health are numerous. Gopal Singh, at the Department of Health and Human Services, along with Mohammad Siahpush, a professor at the University of Nebraska Medical Center, developed an index to measure social and economic conditions using census data on education, income, poverty, housing, and other factors. What they found by examining data from the years 1998 to 2000 was that the affluent live 4.5 years longer than the poor (79.2 years versus 74.7 years). And according to Singh, this longevity gap is widening over time.[32] The affluent are less likely to get almost every disease out there except for cancer, and when they do get cancer, they're much more likely to survive.[33] They are less likely to have accidents or wind up disabled, and their babies are twice as likely to survive as those born into poor families.[34]

Rich people even suffer less than poor people before they die. In one study, researchers interviewed the surviving family members of 2,604 men and women aged 70 or older who had a net worth of $70,000 or more when they died. They found that the individuals with the highest net worth were 33 percent less likely to have suffered from pain in the year before they died. They were also less likely to have experienced depression or shortness of breath. These differences persisted even after researchers took into account the subjects' age, sex, ethnicity, education, and preexisting medical conditions. Why is this so? Researchers postulated that those with greater financial resources may express their symptoms more assertively and demand better care. They may also have greater access to services that health insurance might not cover.[35]

Of course, these disparities pose one of those chicken/egg conundrums. Are rich people able to earn more money because they're healthier? Are poor people financially disadvantaged because they're sick? Or do the wealthy just have access to better preventive health and exotic treatments because they can afford to pay for them?

You might argue that access to premium health care explains the divide, but studies show this is not the case. When offered the same health insurance benefits, people higher up in a company's pecking order are still healthier than those lower down.[36] Some health officials believe it's because social inequality itself is the killer. People of lower socioeconomic status may feel like they have less control over their lives and worry more about their basic needs, which activates the body's stress response.

You might be stressed because you just declared bankruptcy, your stocks went down, you got demoted, you're unemployed, or you can't afford to get food on the table. But even if none of these things are true, you could still be stressed at the very *idea* of them. The body can't differentiate between perceived financial stress (fear that you'll wind up flat broke) and real financial stress (you *really are* flat broke). Either way, the stress response becomes chronically activated, and this can translate into disease.

But it doesn't have to be this way. While you may not be able to change your financial status overnight, you can change how your mind responds to money worries.

Happy Workers Are Healthy Workers

Unsurprisingly, work environments that avoid shaming employees, encourage creativity, allow flexibility, and foster positive inter-office relationships have also been linked to better employee health. Those with effective employee wellness programs that are linked to financial incentives, such as Safeway, get bonus points for improving health outcomes in their workers.[37] But it's not just about making sure the workplace avoids shame and chooses healthy food for the cafeteria. There's also evidence that, while work stress can literally kill you, doing work you love just might save your life.[38]

Finding your professional bliss can be medicine for the mind, and the body responds with better health and more happiness. Happiness researcher Sonja Lyubomirsky, author of *The How of Happiness*, asserts that people who strive for something significant personally and professionally are happier than those who don't have strong dreams and aspirations. She says, "Find a happy person, and you will find a project."

Studies show that the process of working toward a goal and participating in challenging and stimulating work experiences is as important as actually achieving what it is you desire.[39] Committed pursuit of goals gives us a sense of mission, of pursuit, of being part of something bigger than ourselves, and studies show that this increases our sense of control over our lives, which is known to affect the health of the body.[40]

When your work involves pursuing goals that are personally resonant for you, it boosts your self-esteem as you start checking off the baby-step goals that get you closer to your big dream; it lifts you up and motivates you to keep on plugging away, doing what you love, even when the pursuit of these goals may require tedious tasks, risk-taking, and uncertainty. Pursuing goals also adds meaning and structure to our lives, keeping us on task, ensuring that the world will be a better place because we were in it. Striving to leave a legacy or pursue a calling increases happiness, which leaves the body flooded with health-inducing hormones that strengthen the immune system, relax the cardiovascular system, and deactivate the stress response.

Keep in mind that when I talk about "work," I'm talking about whatever you spend the majority of your day doing. For some, this is a paid position. Others might not get paid, but still work their butts off raising children, caring for ailing parents, or volunteering, and these jobs can be every bit as stressful as any paid profession, with equally negative effects on the body. They can also bring just as much meaning and purpose to your life, resulting in positive effects on the body. In fact, finding meaning in your work strongly protects you from burnout. In his research on physician burnout, burnout researcher and Stanford professor Tait Shanafelt, M.D., found that most people vacillate in their experience of the work they do. Sometimes it feels like a job, something you do just to earn a paycheck. Other times it feels like a career, a way to earn your way up the ladder and achieve certain ambitions. But sometimes the work takes on a quality of sacredness that makes it feel like a calling. Shanafelt found that if you are doing something personally meaningful, perceiving your work as a calling at least 20 percent of the time, this tends to protect you from burnout, even if you're doing stressful work over long hours.[41] In other words, meaning is the medicine that can help protect you from some of the negative health effects of work life.

The key is to remember that how our minds feel as we go about our day—how relaxed, happy, and fulfilled we are—gets translated into the physiology of the body. Way too many people subscribe to the TGIF mentality that leads them to dread Mondays, breathe a sigh of relief on hump day, and then drink way too much all weekend before putting their heads down and grinding away again at a job they don't enjoy. Or they quit a job they love to stay home with the kids, only to resent what they gave up, which leads to its own kind of stress.

However, when you feel free to be creative in your work, enjoy autonomy and respect, have clear goals and measures of achievement, are well supported by your co-workers, believe that your work is in line with your integrity, know that what you're doing helps other people, have a sense of mission, purpose, and meaning, express your unique gifts in your work, get paid well, and spend enough time away from your work to pursue other activities, you're less likely to experience work stress and more likely to be optimally healthy.

Creativity and Health

Creativity may seem like a peripheral factor in your health. Who ever heard of prescribing a hobby as preventive medicine or treatment for a disease? But scientific evidence shows that creative expression can elicit relaxation responses that counterbalance stress responses. In fact, artist Shiloh Sophia, who has been recognized by and presented to the United Nations, uses a painting process called "intentional creativity" to treat mental and physical illness in women who have experienced trauma.

Sadly, being creative gets a bad rap in our society. From the time we're children, we are indoctrinated into thinking that science, math, and business are more valuable than art, music, theater, and writing. What our society seems to have forgotten is that being creative is not only fun; it's also good for your health. Keep in mind that when I talk about expressing yourself creatively, I use a very loose definition of the word "creativity." I'm not limiting creativity to the arts. In some cases, your form of creative expression might be painting, dancing, playing an instrument, or writing poetry. But you may also express your creativity by scrapbooking, flower arranging, photography, gardening, interior decorating, blogging, knitting, hula-hoop dancing, singing in the shower, or brainstorming business ideas. You might express yourself by cooking a gourmet meal, crafting music playlists, salsa dancing, or generating ideas for new products at work. You might create workshops, design jewelry, or bake the perfect cupcake.

Whatever you do, flexing your creative muscles is as important to overall health and happiness as flexing your biceps. The link between creativity and health has been well established, so anything that allows you to be more creative in your life benefits the physiology of your body and mind.[42] Creative expression releases endorphins and other feel-good neurotransmitters, reduces depression and anxiety, improves your immune function, relieves physical pain, and activates the parasympathetic nervous system, thereby lowering your heart rate, decreasing your blood pressure, slowing down your breathing, and lowering cortisol.

Health benefits of creative expression include improved sleep, better overall health, fewer doctor visits, less use of medication, and fewer vision problems. Creativity decreases symptoms of distress and improves quality of life for women with cancer; it strengthens positive feelings, alleviates distress, and helps clarify existential and spiritual issues; it lowers the risk of Alzheimer's disease, reduces anxiety, and improves mood, social functioning, and self-esteem.[43]

When we unleash the creative process, we tap into subconscious processes that help us heal—and thrive. Expressing yourself creatively exercises the right side of your brain, and doing so not only affects the body—it also affects your emotional state, leading to greater happiness. And as we'll discuss in Chapter 7, it's a well-documented phenomenon that happy people are more likely to be healthy.

The health benefits of creativity are incredible—and that's just how creative expression affects the individual! Creativity also affects your work life, your relationships, your sexuality, your spirituality, and your mental health. As art therapist Marti Hand teaches, expressing yourself creatively also promotes social peace by enhancing compassion, tolerance, kindness, harmony, expansion, growth, collaboration, respect, and healing. Even seemingly unrelated benefits may arise as the result of expressing yourself creatively, such as improved fertility.

While your creative life can be a potent source of physiological relaxation, it can also be a stressor if you're feeling creatively thwarted. One of my patients had been writing a novel in her head for years, but because she was so busy at work, her novel went unwritten. Every day, she felt stressed about the fact that she might die one day without ever writing her book. Creativity only heals you if you make the time to prioritize it. So don't forget about expressing yourself in your own way.

We all have a song within us longing to be sung as only we can sing it. As poet Mary Oliver writes, "Tell me, what is it you plan to do with your one wild and precious life?"

Finding Your Calling

At 59 years old, Andy Mackie had undergone nine heart surgeries and was taking 15 medications to try to keep himself alive, but he was so sick from the side effects of the drugs that he'd finally had enough. He announced to his doctors that he was stopping all his drugs, which worried his medical team, who insisted that he would die within a year if he quit his medications. Andy was prepared to die, but since the three things he valued in life were love, family, and music, he decided to go out making music. Since he figured he had nothing to lose, he decided to indulge a lifelong dream: He chose to spend the money he had been spending on medications buying 300 harmonicas for kids in the local public school, and he volunteered to give them harmonica lessons himself. He believed everyone can learn to play an instrument and that doing so leads to greater happiness. So he committed himself to helping leave a few kids lit up because of his musical influence on them. The following month, Andy was still alive and kicking, feeling better off of all those drugs, so he bought another 300 harmonicas. Time passed, and he still hadn't died, so he started the Andy Mackie Music Foundation, which supplies instruments and music lessons to children. His foundation even taught them how to make their own instruments and funds college music scholarships. Thirteen years, 20,000 harmonicas, and 5,500 "Mackie Music Sticks" later, Andy Mackie finally passed away.

For many years I've been collecting stories like Andy's, marveling at people who are supposed to die but live extended lives after finding service-oriented work or an unpaid passion project that calls to them from deep in their hearts. As I wrote in my book *The Anatomy of a Calling* and touched on at the beginning of this book, I was once sick and depressed in a job that was sucking the life out of me. On the fast track to either a heart attack or suicide, my path to optimal health required me to leave a respected, well-paid profession most people don't dare to leave. But like Andy Mackie, I too got excited about work I'm passionate about. Once saddled with seven drugs that my doctors told me I would need my whole life, I was off all of them within two years of leaving the hospital and feeling better than ever 12 years later.

I am not alone. Many people find that the best medicine is finding meaningful work that allows you to give away your true gifts and have them received by the people who appreciate and benefit from them. Finding meaning in your work and allowing yourself to lean into the gratitude that comes with feeling fulfilled by your work creates the biochemistry of healing, disabling stress responses and filling your body with the hormones of love and restoration. For some people, changing careers to fulfill a calling can be the most potent medicine on the planet.

Rx for Job Stress

If you're feeling stressed about work or money, don't despair. You don't necessarily have to turn in your resignation letter or win the lottery in order to counteract the stress response. But you do have to have a serious heart-to-heart with yourself about how these issues might be affecting your health.

If you're committed to preventing disease or healing yourself from illness, be brave enough to tell yourself the truth. If you're concerned about how these stressors might be affecting your body, all is not lost. There's hope. You may be able to prevent disease or reverse illness by making positive changes aimed at bringing more relaxation into your body. If you're powerless to change your professional life, you still have the power to change how you react to stressful situations at work. You can learn to stand up for yourself, set clear boundaries, limit your hours, turn off your gadgets when you go home, and make clear requests about how you might get your needs met at work. You might be surprised at how quickly some employers will bend over backward to meet your needs once they realize they might lose you. You can also be proactive about focusing on the sacredness and meaning in the work you're privileged to do, no matter how modest your work might seem. You can also counteract at least a percentage of the negative effects of the stress response on your body with techniques clinically proven to activate the body's physiological relaxation response and improve your health. (I'll be discussing these health-inducing techniques in Chapter 8.)

Until then, know this: stripping off the masks we wear in order to impress other people, appear more "professional," cover up our imperfections, and protect ourselves from getting hurt can work wonders when we're on a quest for optimal health. Being unapologetically who we are—not just at work but at home, in the schoolyard, at church, wherever—soothes the mind, halts the stress response, induces the relaxation response, and heals the body. Authenticity, in work and in life, as well as meaning, service, and the fulfillment of expressing a true calling, can be medicine for the body.

CHAPTER 7

HAPPINESS IS PREVENTIVE MEDICINE

Happiness is not something ready made.
It comes from your own actions.

— HIS HOLINESS THE DALAI LAMA

It may seem obvious that happy, well-adjusted people are health-ier. But when was the last time your doctor prescribed a program to learn optimism as a tool for preventing heart disease as effective as smoking cessation? When have you ever prescribed for yourself, as part of your preventive medicine regimen, lifestyle modifications and practices scientifically proven to increase your happiness as a way of extending your life by 7 ½ to 10 years? Has anyone ever suggested that treating—and really clearing—your trauma in order to make joy more accessible to you might have far more impact on your likelihood of radical remission than any medical prescription?

In modern medicine, emotional and mental health often take a backseat to biochemically rooted physical health concerns. We tend to relegate emotional and mental health to the dark recesses of psychiatrists' offices, focusing instead on more physical pre-ventive-health measures, such as a healthy diet, exercise, smoking cessation, and weight management. But the scientific data linking happiness and health is shocking enough that it just might convince you that treatments aimed at increasing happiness, along with hap-piness's twin sister, optimism, should take center stage when you're interested in preventing disease.

Multiple studies show that happiness and health are inextricably linked.[1] Sure, we all know that those who suffer from mental health conditions such as depression, anxiety, or bipolar disorder are at increased risk of suicide, substance abuse, and other life-threatening conditions that directly affect the health of the body. But it might surprise you to know you don't have to experience full-blown mental health disorders that meet DSM-5 criteria for generalized anxiety disorder or major depression to have your mood affect your health. There's nothing wrong with feeling any human emotion. All emotions are meant to arise and move through you relatively quickly. But when feelings like anxiety, sadness, anger, helplessness, frustration, or hopelessness get repressed, these stuck emotional energies, often caused by unhealed traumas, can make us sick.

Surveys of U.S. adults show that just over half (54 percent) rate themselves as "moderately mentally healthy" but not exactly flourishing.[2] Depression affects more than 21 million Americans annually and 300 million people globally and is the leading cause of disability in the United States for individuals ages 15 to 44. It is also the principal cause of 30,000 suicides in the U.S. each year.[3] Twenty-one percent of Americans will suffer from a mood disorder such as depression in their lifetime, 28 percent will suffer from an anxiety disorder, and one in five Americans takes psychiatric medications, mostly antidepressants.[4]

Anxiety is an epidemic as well, with 40 million Americans and 300 million people worldwide suffering from anxiety disorders. As I reported in my book *The Fear Cure*, "Fear tends to masquerade as a lot of other emotions. Perhaps because the word *stress* refers more to a physical reaction than to an emotion, we seem to be more willing to admit that *stress* is what plagues us, rather than worry, anxiety, or fear. In fact, for many, being stressed out is practically a badge of honor. We parade our stress as proof that we're busy, productive, valuable people leaving our mark on the world. But for many people, being 'stressed out' is just the code word for being really, really scared."

The problem is not that anxious people feel fear. All emotions are welcome and are here to help you, including fear and anxiety. The challenge lies in getting stuck in anxiety loops, which are almost always the result of unhealed trauma. Such ruminating, anxious thoughts stimulate chronic repetitive stress responses that predispose the body to disease. According to the scientific data I quoted in *The Fear Cure*, anxiety has been scientifically linked to heart disease, cancer, immune dysfunction, the common cold, and many chronic diseases.

With one in six Americans—totaling 40 million people—taking daily psychiatric medication, it's clear that our society is not fostering mentally healthy, happy, peaceful lives for many of its citizens. This is nobody's fault. As Charles Eisenstein describes it, depression may be a "mutiny of the soul." He writes:

> When our soul-body is saying No to life, through fatigue or depression, the first thing to ask is, "Is life as I am living it the right life for me right now?" When the soul-body is saying No to participation in the world, the first thing to ask is, "Does the world as it is presented me merit my full participation?"
>
> What if there is something so fundamentally wrong with the world, the lives, and the way of being offered us, that withdrawal is the only sane response? Withdrawal, followed by a reentry into a world, a life, and a way of being wholly different from the one left behind?[5]

If you are feeling such profound withdrawal from business as usual, what might you require to want to fully participate in life again? You may feel powerless right now to change a systemically sick culture that causes many souls to mount a mutiny. But while you're not in control, you do have the power to make change in your life and in the world, to be proactive about living a life your physical and emotional body will love.

Clearly, many people feel mentally unhealthy. But what exactly is happiness, and what does it have to do with the health of the body? Happiness researchers define happiness as "the overall appreciation of one's life-as-a-whole."[6] Essentially, it's a measure of how much you like the life you're living and how much enthusiasm you feel when you wake up every day.

Studies show that positive psychological states, such as joy, happiness, and positive energy, as well as characteristics such as life satisfaction, hopefulness, optimism, and a sense of humor, result in lower mortality rates and extended longevity in both healthy and diseased populations.[7] In fact, happiness and related mental states reduce the risk or limit the severity of heart disease, lung disease, diabetes, hypertension, and colds. According to a Dutch study of elderly patients, upbeat mental states reduced an individual's risk of death by 50 percent over the study's nine-year duration.[8]

The Grant Study

The link between happiness and physical health became apparent during a landmark longitudinal study called the Grant Study, which followed upstanding, exceptionally gifted Harvard sophomores from three classes who were believed to be the pinnacle of physical fitness, mental health, and hope for the future. The goal was to watch how they lived their lives; pay attention to their health, happiness, relationships, and achievements; and hopefully learn how to predict, and thereby potentially control, why some people live happy, healthy, successful lives while others don't.

To choose just the right subjects for the Grant Study, Dr. Arlie Bock's team combed through medical records, academic records, and personal recommendations from the dean. The 268 Harvard students, mostly from the classes of 1942, '43, and '44, underwent evaluation by psychologists, social workers, physiologists, doctors, and pretty much everyone else Bock could assemble to record data about who these young men were as college sophomores.

Comprehensive medical examinations noted everything from organ function to the hanging length of the scrotum to brain activity as measured by electroencephalography. Social workers recorded bed-wetting habits, how the subjects received sex ed, and the family dynamics of their youth. The young men interpreted Rorschach inkblots, got their handwriting analyzed, and submitted to extensive psychiatric evaluation. All were deemed "normal," even "gifted."

The young men then graduated from college, but Bock, and those who took over for him over the years, studied them for the rest of their lives. The men were followed with extensive physical checkups, periodic interviews, and questionnaires, producing a veritable gold mine of information about what makes a person healthy, happy, and successful in life.

As the young men went off to fight in the wars that followed graduation from college, many of them endured the traumas that accompany combat. In spite of the challenges they faced, though, many of the men became quite successful. Four of them ran for U.S. Senate. One was a best-selling novelist, one became the editor of *The Washington Post*, one was a Cabinet member, and one even became president. (It was later revealed that one of the Grant Study participants was John F. Kennedy.)

But as time went on, a trend began to emerge. By 1948, 20 of the young men displayed signs of severe psychiatric illness. By the time they turned 50, a third of them were mentally ill. Turns out that beneath the promising veneer of hopeful dean's-list sophomores lurked unexpected turmoil.

As quoted in an article in *The Atlantic*, Bock said, "They were normal when I picked them. It must have been the psychiatrists who screwed them up."[9]

Depression in these men turned out to be strongly linked to physical health. Of those diagnosed with depression by age 50, more than 70 percent had died or were chronically ill by 63. Those who reported being extremely satisfied with their lives had one-tenth the rate of severe illness or death compared to their unhappy counterparts. These findings held up after screening out other contributing factors, such as alcohol, tobacco, obesity, and ancestral longevity.[10]

Are Optimists Healthier than Pessimists?

Many years later, Martin Seligman, the father of positive psychology and author of *Learned Optimism*, was seeking a way to study whether optimists live longer than pessimists. For many years, he had been researching people's explanatory styles, how they explain unfortunate or fortunate events in their lives. As it turns out, the difference between optimists and pessimists lies in how permanent, pervasive, and personal they perceive good and bad events to be.

Because the pessimist views the bad event as permanent ("It'll always be this bad"), pervasive ("This is going to ruin everything"), and personal ("It's all my fault"), hopelessness ensues. When you make permanent, pervasive, and personal explanations for the painful events that inevitably happen to everyone, you pave the way for chronic unhappiness and, ultimately, illness. Pessimists also believe that events they judge as bad are the result of their own failure. Good events, on the other hand, they believe to be temporary, specific, and outside of their control. Optimists, meanwhile, are a whole different breed. Optimists perceive bad events to be temporary, specific, and external, while they believe good events are permanent, pervasive, and the result of their own internal awesomeness.

Seligman and his colleagues sought out the Grant Study data to see if they could identify any correlations between explanatory style and disease risk. First, they had to determine whether optimism and pessimism are stable across a lifetime. Is it "once an optimist, always an optimist"? Or do people change?

What they found is that, while optimism may change over time, the way people explain painful life events tends to remain fixed throughout their lives unless something significant changes and someone shifts explanatory styles. I'll discuss what you can do to become more optimistic and enjoy the health benefits that accompany optimism at the end of this chapter.

To see if trends in explanatory styles could be linked to health outcomes, Seligman and his partner, Chris Peterson, took a crack at the Grant Study data. What they found was that by the age of 45, the Grant Study pessimists were already less healthy than the optimists. The pessimistic men had started to get sick younger and more severely than the optimistic men. And by the age of 60, pessimists were significantly sicker.[11]

Turns out optimistic patients recover better from coronary bypass surgery, enjoy healthier immune systems, and live longer. They fare better when suffering from conditions such as cancer, heart disease, and kidney failure.[12] Optimists also live longer than pessimists. People with a positive outlook are 45 percent less likely to die within a specified period of time from all causes than negative thinkers (and 77 percent less likely to die from heart disease).[13] A positive attitude also affects our ability to ward off infection. In one study, healthy volunteers were interviewed about attitudes and then exposed to common cold and influenza viruses. Those with sunny dispositions were more resilient than those without.[14]

Other studies examining optimism versus pessimism followed. Harvard psychologist Laura Kubzansky, who studies optimism, tracked 1,300 men for 10 years and found that heart disease rates among optimists were half the rates in pessimists. The difference between the two groups was as dramatic as that seen between smokers and nonsmokers.[15]

As it turns out, pessimists are more susceptible to depression, more likely to experience barriers to professional success, less likely to experience pleasure, more likely to endure challenges in their relationships, and more likely to get sick.[16] Studies show that optimists catch fewer infectious diseases than pessimists, have stronger immune systems and lower blood pressures, live longer, and are less likely to suffer from cardiac disease.[17] In one study, pessimists had twice as many infectious diseases and twice as many doctor visits as optimists.[18]

A sense of positive well-being has been proven to protect your heart. Patients with high levels of "emotional vitality" were 19 percent less likely to develop coronary heart disease than those with lower levels.[19] And just to ice the cake, people with high self-esteem, who view themselves in a more positive light, have lower cardiovascular responses to stress, recover faster, and have lower baseline levels of the stress hormone cortisol.[20]

Hope Heals

When I was a medical student, I took care of a little boy named Joe who had stage 4 cancer. Joe, who had never met his father, was in the middle of aggressive chemotherapy when he wrote a pleading letter telling his father how sick he was and begging him to fly to

Florida so they could meet. Knowing the man's whereabouts, his mother promised to send the letter, and to Joe's delight, his father wrote back and promised to come see him in the hospital—for the first time in his life.

As he waited for the visit from his father, Joe's cancer wasn't responding well to the treatment. His body was becoming progressively weaker. But Joe was an optimist. He believed he would recover from the cancer and have the rest of his long life to finally get to know his father, whom he had been fantasizing about for as long as he could remember.

At one point, Joe's organs began to shut down, and we were sure the end was near. His mother called his father to tell him to come quickly, and that night, Joe got word that his father had bought his plane ticket and would be arriving in a week. By the next day, Joe's condition had significantly improved, and he was up, walking around the ward, excitedly telling all the nurses about his father's impending visit.

The reunion was to happen on a Saturday. Joe spent the whole week making drawings for his father, writing stories, and practicing a song on his recorder to play for him. We were amazed at how sprightly Joe suddenly appeared, in anticipation of his father's visit.

Friday night, Joe couldn't sleep. My attending physician finally ordered a sleeping pill so Joe wouldn't be completely exhausted when his father arrived. Saturday morning, Joe begged us to let him out of the hospital so he could go to the airport and see his father the moment he walked off the plane. But Joe still needed his IV, and the doctor wouldn't let him go. Instead, Joe camped out on the front patio of the hospital in a wheelchair with his IV pole, where he waited with his mother and watched for the taxi that would bring his father to the hospital.

His father's plane was to arrive at 2:00. The airport wasn't far. He should have been there no later than 3:30. But 3:30 came and went. Joe waited. And waited. And waited. But his father never came. His mother called, but nobody picked up. Joe left messages, but nobody ever called back.

I was working that day, and I kept checking on Joe, who insisted his father's plane had been delayed or he was just stuck in traffic.

But his mother had checked the flight. It had arrived right on schedule. Joe's mother tried to explain to him that his father wasn't very mature and didn't quite know how to be a father. But Joe wasn't buying it. He was certain his father was coming. Nothing could shake his faith.

I was on call that night, worried about Joe but running around, taking care of new admissions to the pediatric ward, when finally, at 11 P.M., eight hours after his father was supposed to arrive, Joe's mom was able to convince him to return to his room. When I saw Joe's wheelchair rolling through the halls and leaned in to hug him, Joe started crying and told me his father had stood him up. The whole ward—me, the nurses, Joe's mom—got misty-eyed as we watched Joe's thin little body shake with sobs.

Sometime around midnight, Joe finally fell asleep.

About five hours later, when I was still in the emergency room, writing up another history and physical exam as I admitted a baby with meningitis, the overhead speaker blared, "Ninety-nine, Doctor Heart," our secret code for a code blue. Someone was dying, and as the medical student on call, it was my job to be there. When I called the operator to find out where the code was happening, she gave me the room number.

My own heart almost stopped when I realized it was Joe's room.

Although he had been doing well the night before, Joe stopped breathing, and our resuscitation efforts failed. Joe's dad never came, even when Joe's mother reluctantly invited him to the funeral.

You might say that hope had been keeping Joe alive—that's how powerful the effect of optimism can be. But while Joe's story of hope withdrawn has a sad ending, Maria's story of how hope heals has a happy one. Maria was eight when she was diagnosed with a form of leukemia for which her doctors recommended toxic doses of chemotherapy, followed by a bone marrow transplant. However, a transplant match couldn't be found. So Maria's parents made the radical choice to conceive a baby, hoping that the sibling would be a match.

While Maria's mother was pregnant, Maria's doctors treated Maria with lower doses of chemotherapy, which they believed would keep the leukemia in check but not cure her. The goal was to keep her alive until the baby was born, when cord blood collected at the time of birth could be screened and, they hoped, used for transplantation.

Maria, who had always wanted a sibling, was overjoyed that her mother was pregnant. Although the chemotherapy weakened her, her spirits stayed high, and she told all the nurses that her cancer was going away so she could be a good big sister. Not wanting to remove hope or interfere with her optimism, the nurses nodded in agreement, even though the blood tests revealed that the cancer was still there.

Maria tolerated the chemotherapy well, and a few months later, to the surprise of her doctors, her blood counts started to improve beyond what they had expected with the low doses of chemotherapy they were using.

When the baby was born, Maria was in the room, outfitted with gear meant to protect her frail, susceptible body from infection. When she rocked her new sister in her arms, those present at the delivery were deeply moved.

But the cord blood collected at the time of delivery was not a close enough match for Maria. Maria's parents were devastated, but Maria told them not to worry, that her cancer had gone away and she didn't need the bone marrow transplant anymore. Her oncologists shook their heads. That would be impossible, they said. The doses of chemotherapy she had received were insufficient to result in cure.

But it turned out Maria was right. During her next round of tests, no trace of her cancer could be found. Although some might argue that the low doses of chemotherapy cured her, what if hope and optimism did?

Learned Helplessness and Illness

When you work in a hospital, you often hear inspiring stories of optimism linked to disease remission and pessimism associated with disease progression. Martin Seligman claims that what differentiates the pessimists from the optimists is something he calls "learned helplessness." When things don't go the way we hope, we all—optimists and pessimists alike—feel temporarily helpless.

When your boyfriend breaks up with you, your boss hands you your pink slip, your wife dies, your child is kidnapped, or you get slapped with a cancer diagnosis, you get the proverbial wind knocked out of you, and you're likely to experience negative emotions like sadness, anger, worry, grief, and fear.

When bad things happen, however, the difference between optimists and pessimists is that optimists start to recover right away. Something in them knows they'll always land butter side up, even when they're in the thick of it. Optimists might feel demoralized, even temporarily depressed, but they pick themselves up, brush themselves off, and get back to the business of living a happy life.

Pessimists, on the other hand, continue to feel helpless over an extended period of time, which often spirals downward into full-blown clinical depression. Studies show that when pessimists fail—in relationships, in business, in the achievement of personal goals—they feel helpless, since it feels like the negative experience will last forever, will ruin everything, and has come about as the result of internal personal failure. Over time, they learn helplessness that leaves them feeling in the dumps, often for a long, long time.[21] We've long known that negative thoughts and stressors can make us sick, and researchers suspect that negative belief affects the body by triggering the stress response, turning off the body's natural self-repair mechanisms and predisposing the body to disease.[22]

Immune Response and Helplessness

On a mission to further elucidate the mechanism by which helplessness might be linked to illness, Madelon Visintainer, a colleague of Seligman's, performed a study on three groups of rats. The first group was given a mild, escapable shock—one the rats could avoid once they learned how. The second group was given a mild, inescapable shock, which rendered them helpless. The third group was given no shock at all.

Before setting about shocking these poor rats, Visintainer implanted a few cancer cells on each rat's flank. The cancer was the kind that would invariably kill the rat if the rat's immune system failed to fend it off. Visintainer carefully controlled the number of cancer cells she implanted so she could expect that, under normal conditions, about half the rats would reject the tumor and live. The other half would succumb and die.

Everything external was perfectly controlled—the rats' diet, how they were housed, the tumor burden. The only difference between the three groups of rats was their psychological experience. The rats experiencing escapable shocks quickly learned how to game the system, ultimately avoiding the shocks. The rats getting inescapable shocks, on the other hand, were learning helplessness. And the unshocked rats were just minding their own business, with neither the challenge of figuring something out nor the trauma of getting shocked.

As expected, within a month, 50 percent of the unshocked rats had died, while the other 50 percent of unshocked rats fought off the tumor. But curiously, the rats given escapable shocks, who learned how to master the system, rejected the tumor 70 percent of the time, giving them a survival advantage over the unshocked rats. The rats who couldn't escape the shocks, however, wound up listless and helpless, and only 27 percent rejected the tumor.[23] From these rats, we may conclude that our sense of control, ability to avoid victimhood, and feelings of hopefulness regarding our experiences, particularly the traumas we face, may affect whether we get sick or stay healthy.

Based on this data, researchers concluded that learned helplessness in rats who couldn't escape the shocks must have suppressed the immune response known to fight off cancer cells in tumors of this sort. Further study of these helpless rats found that, indeed, inescapable shocks weaken the immune system. The T-cells of the helpless rats no longer multiplied or got down to the business of fighting off cancer cells when they came across invading outsiders. Natural killer cells, also important in fighting off cancers and other foreign invaders, lost their natural killer abilities. These studies confirmed what researchers had suspected: psychological states can directly affect the outcome of remission from some diseases, at least those that are immune-mediated, as many cancers are.[24]

This may explain why optimists are healthier than pessimists. Because of their healthier explanatory styles in the face of negative life events, optimists are more likely to learn healthy adaptations in response to life's shocks, making them immune to states of helplessness. Pessimists, on the other hand, feel like life's shocks are inescapable, and like the listless, helpless rats, they get depressed and their immune systems weaken. Over the course of a lifetime, fewer episodes of learned helplessness may keep the immune system stronger, reduce stress responses and their negative health outcomes, and reduce the likelihood of disease.

Control as an Antidote to Helplessness

If rats can fight off cancer by exerting more control over their surroundings, is there any proof that humans respond the same way? Curious as to whether learned helplessness could be counteracted by increasing feelings of control, choice, and personal responsibility, researchers working with residents of a nursing home designed a study to evaluate the physical health of residents in response to positive changes made in the facility.

They divided the home into two groups—the first floor and the second. All residents would be able to enjoy the new benefits the home was offering—omelets versus scrambled eggs, movie night on Wednesdays or Thursdays, plants to enjoy in their own rooms if they wanted them. But in order to take advantage of these opportunities, first-floor residents were given extra choice and extra responsibility: they had to choose which eggs they wanted, sign up for Wednesdays versus Thursdays, and water their own plants.

Second-floor residents, on the other hand, were given the same opportunities, but they were offered no choices or personal responsibilities. Their schedules were set, leaving them essentially powerless. Mondays, Wednesdays, and Fridays were omelet days. Tuesdays and Thursdays were scrambled-egg days. They were assigned a movie night without being given a choice. And they didn't have to pick out or water their own plants.

A year and a half later, researchers found that the first-floor residents, the ones with choice and personal responsibility, were more active, happier, and less likely to have died during the study period.[25] As it turns out, choice, personal responsibility, and the ability to feel useful are good for your health, most likely because you feel happier and this leaves the body better able to repair itself.

In everyday life, being in control and being out of control live in paradox with each other. It's true that we can be proactive, taking charge of our health and doing our best to become health outliers. It's also true that uncertainty is part of life, and life will eventually prove to you that you're not really in control of an uncontrollable universe. Empowerment is a big step up from helplessness, but there are limits to our personal power. The good news is that there is no limit to the mysterious spiritual powers that we can call upon to help us heal. When we surrender to what is, accepting reality and not resisting it, rather than trying to control it, the nervous system relaxes into a state of trusting life, and this can activate the body's self-repair mechanisms and positively impact health.

Cheerfulness Predicts Longevity

We know that unhappy people are less likely to eat well, exercise, and enjoy healthy sleep patterns. But the health consequences of unhappiness aren't explained solely by whether or not unhappy people neglect to care for their bodies. In 1986, David Snowdon began another longitudinal study like the Grant Study, but this time, instead of studying Harvard sophomores, it studied Roman Catholic nuns.

Typically, studying what makes people live longer is fraught with bias. For example, we know that people from Utah live longer than people from Nevada. But why? Is it because the ascetic Mormon lifestyle is healthier than the rough-and-tumble boozing, gambling, and smoking culture of Las Vegas and Reno? Do the people of Utah eat more nourishing foods? Is the air in Utah cleaner? Are Utah residents less stressed?

Because these kinds of variables make longevity studies tough to interpret, it's helpful to study populations for whom many of these variables are controlled. This is where the nun study comes in handy.

The health habits of these nuns were otherwise fairly well controlled—they ate roughly the same bland diet, they didn't smoke or drink, they didn't get married, have babies, or contract sexually transmitted diseases, their social and economic class was similar, and they all had the same access to good medical care. This made it easier to draw conclusions about what leads to a longer life. You'd think that such a similar population might have similar life expectancies, yet with all the typical confounding variables controlled, there was still wide variation in how long the nuns lived and how healthy they were.

Why the disparity? Upon joining the convent, new nuns were asked to write the story of their lives up until that point (the average age of those who wrote these autobiographies was 22). By the time the study began, many of these nuns were already senior citizens. The autobiographies they had written many years earlier were used to assess their happiness in young life. From there on, the nuns were followed for the rest of their lifetimes.

One such sister was Cecilia O'Payne, who became a novice at the School Sisters of Notre Dame in 1932. In her autobiography, she wrote, "God started my life off well by bestowing upon me grace of inestimable value. . . . The past year which I have spent as a candidate studying at Notre Dame College has been a very happy one. Now I look forward with eager joy to receiving the Holy Habit of Our Lady and to a life of union with Love Divine."

By contrast, another nun taking the same vows, Marguerite Donnelly, wrote, "I was born on September 26, 1909, the eldest of seven children, five girls and two boys. . . . My candidate year was spent in the Motherhouse, teaching Chemistry and Second Year Latin at Notre Dame Institute. With God's grace, I intend to do my best for our Order, for the spread of religion and for my personal sanctification."

Can you spot the difference between the two? Cecilia used effervescent words like "very happy" and "eager joy," while Marguerite's prose contained no such cheerfulness.

So what became of these young nuns? As reported in Martin Seligman's book *Authentic Happiness*, at 98 years old, Cecilia O'Payne was reportedly still alive and hadn't been sick a day in her life. Marguerite Donnelly, on the other hand, had a stroke at 59 and died soon afterward.[26]

When researchers investigated the life stories of the nuns, they found that 90 percent of the most cheerful nuns were still alive at age 84, compared to only 34 percent of the least cheerful. In fact, 54 percent of the most cheerful nuns were still alive and kicking it at age 94, compared to 11 percent of the least cheerful. In general, happy nuns were found to live seven and a half years longer than their unhappy counterparts.[27] Other studies show that happy people live up to 10 years longer than unhappy people.[28] Clearly, happiness is preventive medicine, and at the end of this chapter, we'll discuss how you can increase your happiness to assist your body's healing process.

The Physiology of Mood

So what happens to the body when the mind is in a dark place? Emotional suffering might seem to start as thoughts in the mind, but it is ultimately an embodied experience. You don't just experience unhappiness in your mind. You feel it in your body, as suffering cascades through your body via the stress response. When something hurts emotionally, an alarm is sounded. The stress response is triggered, even though there is no immediate bodily threat—just anger, disappointment, frustration, pessimism, heartbreak, grief, and other upsetting emotions. In this next section, we'll discuss the physiology of how anxiety and depression negatively affect the body and how happiness can heal it.

Anxiety

The amygdala, an almond-shaped group of nuclei located in the limbic system, deep within the medial temporal lobes of the brain, is the boss when it comes to processing and storing memories of various emotions. In fact, the amygdala experiences emotions even before the conscious brain does. Repetitive triggering of the stress response makes the amygdala more reactive to apparent threats, which stimulates the stress response, thereby further triggering the amygdala, on and on and on in a vicious cycle. The amygdala serves to help form "implicit memories," traces of past experiences that lie beneath conscious recognition. As the amygdala becomes more sensitized, it increasingly tinges those implicit memories with heightened residues of fear, causing the brain to experience ongoing anxiety that no longer has anything to do with the circumstances at hand.

At the same time, the hippocampus, which is critical for developing "explicit memories"—clear, conscious records of what really happened—gets worn down by the body's stress response. Cortisol and other glucocorticoids weaken synapses in the brain and inhibit formation of new ones. When the hippocampus is weakened, it's much harder to produce new neurons and thus make new memories. As a result, the painful, fearful experiences the sensitized amygdala records get programmed into implicit memory, while the weakened hippocampus fails to record new explicit memories.

When this happens, you wind up with no real memory of what set you off to begin with but with a very clear sense that something bad—something *very bad*—is happening. This explains why those who experience trauma can wind up triggered by situations that stimulate the unconscious mind when the conscious mind has no clue what's going on. You wind up feeling unsafe and anxious, without having any clue why.

Depression

Depression also leads to repetitive activation of the stress response, which, in a cyclic fashion, then leads to depressed mood. With all that cortisol floating around as a result of the stress response, norepinephrine, which normally helps you feel alert and energized, gets depleted, leaving you feeling apathetic and distracted. Cortisol also lowers the production of dopamine, which is important for helping you experience pleasurable feelings.

The stress response also reduces serotonin, the most important neurotransmitter responsible for positive mood. When serotonin levels drop, norepinephrine levels drop even further, sending you into a downward spiral.

In addition to triggering the stress response, negative emotions also enhance the production of pro-inflammatory cytokines, leading to inflammation, which has been linked to certain cancers, Alzheimer's disease, arthritis, osteoporosis, and cardiovascular disease. Furthermore, negative feelings can contribute to delayed wound healing and infection.[29]

When negative mental states like pessimism, helplessness, hopelessness, anxiety, and depression prevail, the stress response flips on and stays on, leading to gastrointestinal disorders, greater vulnerability to infections and cancer, heart disease, endocrine disorders, and more.[30] Happy people appear to have stronger immune systems, as demonstrated by the fact that happy people develop about 50 percent more antibodies in response to flu vaccines and mount stronger immune responses.[31]

When you're unhappy, on the other hand, your immune system weakens, a finding that was confirmed by one study of grieving widowers demonstrating that T-cell multiplication slowed down during the grieving process.[32] Differences in immunity were also seen in a study of optimistic versus pessimistic HIV-positive women.[33]

Happiness

While the neuroscience of unhappy mental states has been heavily studied, happiness is less well understood. However, the advent of functional MRI machines, along with electroencephalography, has made it easier to study the science of happiness. From examining study subjects who reportedly feel blissed out, researchers have concluded that happiness appears to be located in the left prefrontal cortex of the brain.

But what activates this part of the brain? And what can we do to get our left prefrontal cortexes more activated? Most likely, the answer has something to do with neurotransmitters like dopamine, oxytocin, endorphins, nitric oxide, and serotonin.

Researchers break down "happiness" into two types of pleasurable feelings—the anticipation of something positive and the sensory pleasure of actually experiencing it. For example, you might feel happy fantasizing about your upcoming beach vacation in Bali, planning how you'll spend the end-of-year bonus you'll get at work if you do a good job, or visualizing the thrill of finally kissing the object of your affection. But you might also feel happy basking in the warm sun with crystalline blue waters lapping around your body, slipping on the new cashmere sweater you just bought with your end-of-year bonus, and caressing the soft lips of your lover as your body awakens with pleasure.

When you feel happy because you're anticipating something exciting, your brain lights up in the area of the nucleus accumbens, the pleasure center of the brain. Activation of this part of the brain is most likely related to the neurotransmitter dopamine, which mediates the transfer of positive emotions between the left prefrontal cortex and the emotional centers in the nucleus accumbens. People with sensitive dopamine receptors tend to have better moods.

Dopamine may be the primary neurotransmitter associated with the kind of happiness you get when you're moving toward a goal and then achieve it, whereas other neurotransmitters may be responsible for other types of happiness, such as feelings of love or the sensations of physical pleasure. For example, oxytocin, the "cuddle hormone," which plays a role in pair bonding and is released when you fall in love or snuggle your child, may explain part of how happiness affects your health. Made in the hypothalamus and secreted by the pituitary gland, oxytocin reduces inflammation by decreasing cytokines. It also indirectly inhibits release of ACTH, thereby downregulating the HPA axis that gets triggered during the stress response. Happy people have been found to have lower levels of cortisol, most likely because happy people feel less stress, fear, anger, and other emotions known to trigger the stress response.

Oxytocin also activates serotonin receptors, lifting mood, and inhibits the amygdala, from which the fear that can trigger the stress response arises.[34] Oxytocin also stimulates the release of endorphins, nature's morphine, which reduce pain and can lead to euphoric feelings such as the "runner's high" some get while exercising. Endorphins, which are released by the pituitary gland during exercise, love, and excitement, trigger dopamine release, which then stimulates the nucleus accumbens and leads to feelings of pleasure. Feelings of sensory pleasure also stimulate the release of nitric oxide, a potent vasodilator, which increases blood flow and is known to be important in protecting certain organs from ischemic damage, which can occur when an organ doesn't get enough blood flow.

Most likely, happiness also affects the immune system, as demonstrated by the tumor-laden rats subjected to escapable and inescapable shocks. Learned helplessness, experienced not just by rats but by pessimists, who tend to be unhappy, makes the immune system more passive, leaving you more susceptible to infection, cancer, and other immune-mediated diseases. Optimists, who tend to be happier, are less prone to learned helplessness, which, over the course of a lifetime, may keep the immune system scrappier. The effect of fewer stress responses on the body, as well as the long-term consequences of a strong immune system, may explain the longevity differences between happy and unhappy people.

Does Happiness Cure Disease?

While copious evidence supports happiness as preventive medicine, predicting longevity in healthy populations,[35] what is less clear is whether happiness can also help treat existing disease. The data is mixed. Some studies show markedly improved disease recovery rates in happy people.[36] One small study, for example, evaluated 34 women suffering from a second bout of cancer at the National Cancer Institute, where they underwent extensive physical and psychological evaluations that included analysis of optimism. Because survival after a second bout of breast cancer is rare, after about a year, most of the women began to die, but a few survived. Who lived longest? The ones who were happiest.[37]

But while some studies suggest that a cheerful attitude and fighting spirit improve survival in sick patients, the data suggests that a positive attitude, while it may prevent disease, isn't always enough to fight disease once it exists.[38] In fact, some argue that the idea of fighting serious illness with happiness is a preposterous illusion that merely leaves the patient feeling blamed.[39] To suggest to sick people that they need to be perpetually cheerful or risk getting sicker seems not only ludicrous but even downright cruel. My understanding of what promotes healing is making room for healthy expression of the full range of human emotions, without repressing or getting stuck in any single emotion, allowing emotions to move like waves that rise, crest, crash, and dissipate. Perpetual cheerfulness is not consistent with living a human life, so while uplifting emotions are definitely good for you, don't get too hung up on which emotions you're feeling. You're likely to cause more stress responses from trying to stuff emotions you valence as "bad" than from just letting them all flow through you.

Why, then, might generally high levels of contentment and happiness prevent disease but often fail to treat it?

It's hard to say, but most likely it's because the beneficial effect of happiness has more to do with the cumulative physiological effects of happiness on the body than with the ability of a happy or optimistic mood alone to cure the body once things have gone south. For example, it's clear that feeling happy can reduce lifetime exposure to the stress response, limiting cardiovascular risk. But once the coronary arteries are already blocked with atherosclerosis, perhaps a positive mood alone just ain't gonna hack it.

Another explanation for the disparity in data is that disease mechanisms vary, and the mechanisms of self-repair in the body also vary. Happiness, for example, has been shown to improve immune function, while learned helplessness weakens it. But for diseases unrelated to immune function, mood may have less of an impact on disease outcome. Although a person's mental state, mood, and attitude can certainly improve quality of life, it's likely that happiness can only take you so far with certain diseases. But since the data is mixed and happiness has other benefits, what have you got to lose by being proactive about taking steps to feel happier?

Rx for Pessimism

If you're a pessimist prone to unhappiness, don't despair. According to happiness researchers, things like optimism and happiness can be learned, and you can enjoy the physical and mental health benefits as a result. In *Learned Optimism*, Martin Seligman teaches an exercise he calls the ABCs—an acronym for Adversity, Belief, and Consequences. When we encounter adversity, we think about the adverse event, and our thoughts are quickly translated into beliefs, which become habitual if we're not mindful of them. These beliefs have consequences that can affect the way we feel and the actions we choose to take. By learning to modulate how we translate adversity into belief and how we act on those beliefs, you can convert your negative thoughts into hopeful ones.

For example, say someone zips into the parking space you were eyeing (Adversity). You get upset and think, *That driver stole my place. That was a rude and selfish thing to do* (Belief). You get angry, roll down your window, and shout at the other driver (Consequences).

Or your best friend hasn't returned your phone calls (Adversity). You explain this by thinking, *I'm always selfish and inconsiderate. No wonder* (Belief). You feel depressed all day (Consequences).

Seligman recommends keeping an ABC diary for a few days to assess how you respond to adverse events. To do this, you have to tap into your internal dialogue and identify the beliefs that arise in the face of adversity. (Remember that beliefs are thoughts, not feelings. Feelings are actually consequences of your thoughts.) Then record the consequences—how you felt or how you acted in response to the beliefs that arose out of the adverse event. After reviewing the beliefs that arise in the face of adversity, pessimists may notice how the beliefs that arise trigger negative emotional states or behaviors, whereas optimists may notice that their beliefs help them overcome adversity quickly.

Here's the kicker. If you naturally tend toward pessimism, you can learn to change the beliefs that arise in the face of adversity, and by changing these beliefs, you can change the consequences and improve your health. Once you are aware of your knee-jerk pessimistic beliefs, Seligman recommends two ways to deal with them: distracting yourself and thinking about something else, or disputing them.

To distract yourself from a pessimistic belief, try what researchers call a "thought-stopping technique" meant to interrupt habitual thought patterns—for example, slamming the palm of your hand against a wall and yelling "STOP!" You can also ring a loud bell, carry around a three-by-five card with the word STOP in large red letters, or wear a rubber band around your wrist and snap it hard to stop the ruminations. Combining such techniques with attention shifting can produce longer-lasting results. When you shout "STOP!" or snap the rubber band, consciously concentrate on something else.

If that doesn't cut it, schedule time later in the day to ruminate on your pessimistic beliefs. Tell yourself, "Stop. I'll think this over later." Or write your thoughts down. Doing so breaks the rumination cycle and lessens the strength of the negative thoughts.

Even more effective than distracting yourself from your negative ruminations is disputing them. To do this, you have to learn how to argue with yourself. Review your pessimistic belief, tap into the wisdom of your wiser, loving, compassionate self, and make a case to prove yourself wrong. For example, if your best friend doesn't return your calls, and your first thought is *She hates me because I'm a terrible friend*, dispute the thought. Argue that she might be busy, that someone else might not have relayed the messages you left on her machine, that she probably meant to call but got distracted, that really she loves you and you're a good friend. In other words, the problem isn't permanent, pervasive, and personal; it's temporary, specific, and external. Based on this new optimistic belief, you can choose new consequences and abort the downward spiral that pessimistic beliefs trigger.

The keys to successfully disputing your negative beliefs include trying to find evidence that your negative belief is false (if it is), considering alternative interpretations of the adverse event other than the pessimistic explanations you've imagined, determining what payoff you may be gaining from such a negative belief, and, if the belief really is true, thinking through the implications of such a belief. Let's return to the best friend who hasn't called you back. After thinking of alternative explanations for why she didn't call, examine why your mind might race straight to negative assumptions. Perhaps you're getting something out of feeling like a neglected victim. Perhaps you cling to your righteous anger when she doesn't call you back, and your payoff is that you get to feel superior.

If the real reason she didn't call you back is that she hates you because you're a terrible friend, what can you learn from this belief? How can you use this belief to learn to be a better friend? You'll ultimately realize that, if this friendship isn't destined to last, you can probably learn something about yourself from the relationship, and chances are good that there's someone else out there just itching for the title of your new BFF.

In other words, try to talk yourself out of your negative belief, and if you can't, let yourself think things through to the worst possible scenario so you realize that, even if it's true, the implications probably aren't the end of the world.

Seligman also recommends distancing yourself from your pessimistic beliefs, realizing that they are just that—beliefs, not facts—and concluding your inner dialogue with an energizing thought, one that lifts you up rather than dragging you down.

Keep in mind that cognitive behavioral therapies such as the ABCs of learned optimism have limited usefulness if pessimism has developed because of untreated trauma in your system. Such approaches rely on cognitive function, essentially arguing with yourself mentally to talk yourself out of your pessimistic beliefs. Yet if pessimism has arisen because of painful events in childhood that cause you to see the glass half empty, the parts of your brain that carry these traumas don't respond to even the most rational mental arguments. These distorted, disease-inducing ways of viewing the world are simply too deeply embedded in your neurology and your cellular makeup for you to achieve permanent transformation from cognitive approaches alone. The good news is that treating and clearing whatever traumas caused the pessimism in the first place can restore natural optimism. Cutting-edge trauma therapies are transforming people's lives and sometimes even facilitating radical remissions.

Rx for Unhappiness

Becoming happier and healthier requires more than simply shifting from pessimistic to optimistic explanations for adverse events. It requires being proactive about rewiring your brain so your brain doesn't buzz away on autopilot into painful ruminations and pessimistic, fearful thoughts. We used to think that some people were simply born with a greater capacity for happiness than others, and if you were one of the unlucky ones born with a genetic set point tending toward unhappiness, then you were kind of hosed. Because of what we now know about neuroplasticity, we understand that this previous conclusion espoused by happiness researchers is part true and part untrue.

Yes, it's true that happiness is related to activity in the left pre-frontal cortex of the brain, probably because this is the area of the brain responsible for keeping negative thoughts at bay. Some of us, researchers concluded, just naturally have more active left prefrontal cortexes. Studies of twins have shown us that we're all predisposed to have a certain type of temperament. Some of us are naturally sunny, while others are inherently melancholy. Researchers once thought that this genetic set point accounted for 50 percent of your capacity for happiness and there was nothing you could do to change this predisposition. The good news is that just as the science of epigenetics has disproven our theories about genetic determinism and shown us that we can change how our genes express themselves by changing our thoughts, beliefs, and feelings. It's also been proven that we can change the activity of our left prefrontal cortex by engaging in practices intended to rewire our neural pathways in ways that make us more susceptible to feeling naturally joyful.

Although you may think changing your life circumstances will make you happier—when you finally meet "the one," get the perfect job, score the deal, hit the bestseller list, get pregnant, or whatever else your heart desires—the work of happiness researcher Sonja Lyubomirsky suggests that life circumstances account for only 10 percent of our happiness. Whether we're healthy or unhealthy, privileged or poor, beautiful or homely, married or single, or facing some sort of painful life event, does affect us—but not as much as you might think.

Why don't life circumstances account for more of our happiness? Because of a powerful force psychologists call "hedonistic adaptation." When you finally attain something you want—the object of your affection, more money, higher status, greater beauty, or some material possession—it makes you happier for a short while. But you quickly return to whatever baseline set point your left prefrontal cortex determines. When good things happen, we get a happiness boost, but it isn't sustainable. For example, newlyweds feel happier, usually for about two years, and then they return to their happiness set point.[40]

But here's the upside! Forty percent of our happiness is unrelated to any sort of happiness set point and not subject to hedonistic adaptation. Scientific studies show that influencing this 40 percent can be as easy as keeping a gratitude journal every night.[41]

In *The How of Happiness*, Sonja Lyubomirsky shares her findings from a study examining happy people. What she found was that the happiest people were not the richest, most beautiful, or most successful. Instead, as it turns out, the golden ticket to happiness lies in adopting certain behaviors that have been scientifically proven to increase happiness. In her study, happy people shared similar traits. They devoted a lot of time to nurturing their relationships with family and friends, were comfortable expressing gratitude for what they had, were the first to lend a helping hand, practiced optimism when imagining their futures, savored life's pleasures and tried to live in the moment, exercised frequently, were deeply committed to lifelong goals and ambitions, and showed poise and strength when facing life's inevitable challenges.

She also found that you can be happier by avoiding overthinking, cutting yourself loose from ruminating thoughts, eliminating social comparisons, taking action to solve problems right when they arise, seeking meaning amid stress, loss, or trauma, practicing forgiveness, engaging in activities that get you "in the flow," smiling more, and making efforts to take care of your body.

The other piece of good news is that we're learning from cutting-edge neuroscientific discoveries that, because of neuroplasticity, what we once believed to be a predetermined genetic set point of happiness can be altered through spiritual practices like meditation, mystical experiences in nature, shamanic rituals, communal dancing, drumming, art-making, and singing. In his book *Bliss Brain: The Neuroscience of Remodeling Your Brain for Resilience, Creativity, and Joy*, psychologist and researcher Dawson Church, Ph.D., unpacks the neuroscience of how we can literally change our brains in ways that make joyful emotions more accessible, not just to monks who meditate in caves in India, but to the everyday person. The latest neuroscience suggests that the best way to change a brain to be wired for happiness is to engage in practices that light up the "enlightenment circuit." The brain of bliss may be less about lighting up the left prefrontal cortex than about turning off the default mode network (DMN), which is the autopilot mode of the brain, responsible for the background noise of ruminations, anxieties, and worries that plague meditators with what spiritual teachers often call "the monkey mind." Because the DMN obsessively focuses on self-referencing thoughts, the "Me, me, me!" thoughts that cause us to grasp for what we want and resist what we don't want, an active DMN can lead to a lot of unhappiness. Certain kinds of spiritual practices, however, shut down the DMN and the self-referencing parts of the prefrontal cortex that cause obsessive and neurotic thoughts. In other words, we quit "selfing," experiencing a subject-object shift that allows us to feel more at one with all things, which can lead to the ecstasy and bliss experienced meditators report.

Lonely people tend to show heightened activity in the parietal lobe, but meditators show reduced activation. Meditators are less likely to feel lonely, even if nobody is around, most likely because this area of the brain is less active and they feel more connected to life at large. Your social support expands to include the animals, plants, earth, ocean, and stars, since your brain now senses your oneness with all things. Meditation also activates the corpus callosum, the bridge between the brain's left and right hemispheres. This heightens intuition, creativity, problem-solving, focus, integrating information, and, yes, happiness. This lights up the anterior cingulate cortex, which is related to empathy. Meditation also activates the emotional regulation centers in the hippocampus, helping us calm turbulent emotions and reducing reactivity. The "fight-or-flight" sentry in the limbic brain, the amygdala, also quiets down with regular spiritual practice.

In *Bliss Brain*, Church explains that certain parts of the brains of adept meditators shrink, while other parts expand:

> The amygdala, the brain's "fire alarm," decreases in volume. In adepts, disuse causes it to atrophy. The control circuits between the prefrontal cortex and the amygdala become bigger. This is important because the stronger the link is, the less reactive you become. The relationship between these circuits and emotional reactivity is so strong that their size actually predicts the degree of a person's reactivity. Even when not faced with an emotional trigger, the amygdalas of adepts are 50 percent quieter. In people who are very stressed, the opposite effect occurs. The amygdala grows in size. The connections between the regions of the prefrontal cortex that control emotions and the amygdala decay, allowing stress signals to proliferate. What's particularly fascinating to me about this control circuit is that information flows both ways. In stressed people, the circuit sends signals from the amygdala to the prefrontal cortex, hijacking the brain's decision-making centers and paralyzing executive function. But adepts hijack the hijacker. They use this same control circuit in reverse. The prefrontal cortex sends signals the other way, curbing the amygdala and shutting down the stress response. The amygdala can also be regulated by the striatum, especially the basal ganglia. They engage with areas of the PFC to extinguish the amygdala's conditioned responses to fear. Once these structures deep in the brain are activated, emotion control becomes easier.

Family therapist Richard Schwartz, Ph.D., founder of a trauma healing psychotherapy called Internal Family Systems (IFS), proposes that the best way to do this is not to try to transcend the self-focused thoughts, which are often protective parts of the personality doing their best to keep us safe, but rather to become intimate with these parts, learning to love, accept, understand, relax, and earn the trust of the parts that make up the monkey mind instead of trying to meditate them into silence. Then, when it's time to meditate, these parts that have come to trust you might be willing to cooperate, stepping aside and letting you tune in to "Self" energy during your meditations. (The IFS model is based on the idea that we are all composed of a multiplicity of parts, that we are not one unified "self" but rather many parts with one Self with a capital *S* as the leader of these parts.) In the IFS model, no parts are demonized, even the ones conventional society might medicate, hospitalize, shame, send to rehab, or imprison. As we develop compassionate relationships with the parts that chatter away in our minds, these parts begin to trust the wise, grounded, compassionate Self within each of us. Then, because we have prioritized these inner relationships, when it's time to meditate, these parts will be more willing to settle down and allow us to experience a calm, stable feeling of bliss that is not so dependent on whether things are going our way or not. Over time, this equanimity moves off the meditation pillow and follows us through life's everyday moments. In this way, meditation and self-love come together to rewire the brain for greater happiness, while healing trauma as a welcome health- and happiness-inducing side effect. When these parts begin to heal and trust the leadership of the Self, our minds become less obsessed with the voices of our "parts" and shift to the selfless state seen in advanced meditators when activity in the prefrontal cortexes on both sides slows down, allowing us to live in a more perpetual state of "bliss brain."

What are the qualities of the "bliss brain"? As cited in *Bliss Brain*, priest, researcher, and professor Andrew Greeley and his colleagues at the National Opinion Research Center at the University of Chicago surveyed 1,467 people to learn more about mystical states of consciousness. Among responders, 39 percent (approximately 600 people) reported the following commonalities:

- Feeling of deep and profound peace (55 percent)
- Certainty that all things will work out for the good (48 percent)
- Sense of my own need to contribute to others (43 percent)
- Conviction that love is at the center of everything (43 percent)
- Sense of joy and laughter (43 percent)
- An experience of greater emotional intensity (38 percent)
- Great increase in my understanding and knowledge (32 percent)
- Sense of the unity of everything and my own part in it (29 percent)
- Sense of new life or living in the world (27 percent)
- Confidence in my own personal survival (27 percent)
- Feeling that I couldn't possibly describe what was happening to me (26 percent)
- The sense that all the universe is alive (25 percent)
- The sensation that my personality has been taken over by something much more powerful than I am (24 percent)
- A sense of tremendous personal expansion, either psychological or physical (22 percent)[42]

In addition to spiritual practices that can rewire your brain as a prescription for more happiness, I believe that living in alignment with your truth is also vital to happiness, and studies confirm this. Steve Cole and his colleagues at UCLA investigated HIV-positive gay men to determine whether how "out" or "closeted" they were with their homosexuality affected their disease progression. Study participants were asked to rate themselves as "definitely in the closet," "in the closet most of the time," "half in and half out," "out most of the time," or "completely out of the closet."

Researchers then followed the course of their disease. What did they find? On all counts, HIV infection advanced more quickly in direct proportion to how "in the closet" the patients were. The more they lived in alignment with their truth, the healthier they were. And the results weren't subtle. Those who were mostly or all the way in the closet hit critically low CD4 counts 40 percent faster than those who were mostly or all the way out, and the closeted men died 21 percent faster.[43]

Of course, everything else we've talked about in this book so far—being part of a healthy community, expressing yourself creatively, being sexually authentic, and finding and fulfilling your calling—can also conspire to raise your happiness quotient and improve your mental health. We'll talk more about how to write The Prescription for a happier life in Part Three. Suffice it to say that when you make efforts to increase your happiness, the health of the body tends to follow.

CHAPTER 8

HOW TO COUNTERACT THE STRESS RESPONSE

You can't heal your body until you've blessed your body.

— ANDREW HARVEY

Although it's common knowledge now, as recently as the 1960s, it was heresy for a doctor to suggest that stress and disease were linked. In fact, nobody linked even diseases like hypertension to stress, even though the word *tension* is part of the diagnosis. Doctors knew that patients tended to run higher blood pressures when they visited the doctor's office—they called it "white coat hypertension." But somehow, nobody thought through the implications of the fact that visiting the doctor can be anxiety-provoking and that such stress resulted in elevations of blood pressure that dropped once the patients went back home and relaxed.

Curious about whether there could be a link between stress and high blood pressure, Harvard cardiologist Dr. Herbert Benson started discussing it with his colleagues, who mostly thought he was wacko for even suggesting it. But Benson was dogged in his pursuit of the answers, and finding none, he started researching the topic himself. Inspired by the work of B. F. Skinner and Neal Miller on biofeedback and its ability to teach the body to control apparently involuntary physiological phenomena, he started rewarding monkeys for increasing and decreasing their own blood pressure. He signaled success to them by flashing colored lights. Eventually, he was able to train the monkeys to control their own blood pressure by simply signaling them with the lights. The monkeys were able to control their blood pressure with nothing more than brainpower alone.

The study, which was published in 1969, caught the attention of practitioners of Transcendental Meditation (TM), which had recently been popularized by the Beatles, Mia Farrow, and other celebrities. These practitioners, who had heard that Benson was studying monkeys, believed they were lowering their blood pressure when they meditated, but nobody had ever tried to prove it. Already on shaky ground at Harvard for wandering into the territory of what would ultimately be called "mind-body medicine," Benson originally refused to do the study. But the meditation advocates were persistent.

He then heard about another researcher, Robert Keith Wallace, who was studying TM for his doctoral dissertation at the University of California, Irvine. The two decided to put their curious heads together and collaborate on a study. Once they compiled the data, they were shocked. The data was incontrovertible. Striking physiological changes accompanied meditation—sharp drops in heart rate, respiratory rate, and metabolic rate. In the initial study, the blood pressures of the study subjects didn't drop during meditation, but overall, the study group that meditated had significantly lower baseline blood pressures than those who didn't.

Benson named the physiological changes that meditating people experienced "the relaxation response," a term I've used throughout this book as the opposite of "the stress response." He argued that like the stress response, triggered when a part of the hypothalamus is stimulated, the relaxation response is flipped on when a different part of the hypothalamus is stimulated, as a safeguard intended to counterbalance the emergency alarm the body sometimes sounds.

Benson was so impressed by the benefits he witnessed when patients practiced this simple technique that he asked himself the question—if a 10- to 20-minute meditation practice could result in such profound health benefits, what would happen with those who practiced advanced meditation? Rumors of seemingly impossible feats of physiological manipulation were swirling around at the time. Researchers who studied meditating monks had demonstrated that they were able to reduce their metabolic rate by 20 percent, something usually achieved only after four or five hours of sleep. This demonstrated that it was possible to manipulate "involuntary" mechanisms in the body exclusively through shifts in consciousness.

When he first approached Tibetan monks, they had no interest in being studied. Then Benson befriended the Dalai Lama, who supported his research. All of a sudden, the monks paid attention. He witnessed the monks, dressed in nothing but loincloths, wrapping themselves in wet sheets in freezing temperatures at 15,000 feet in the Himalayas. But instead of shivering, dropping their body temperatures, and possibly dying, the monks visualized fires in their bellies, raising their body temperatures enough to dry the wet sheets.

Benson realized that the fertile breeding ground of the relaxation response might be harnessed to implant thoughts in the mind by visualizing an outcome you wish to achieve—such as raising your body temperature, lowering your blood pressure, healing your cancer, or alleviating back pain. He went on to study processes like these throughout his extensive career as a researcher. Over the years, Benson studied thousands of patients and published scores of articles in scholarly medical journals. Through this research, he elucidated a list of the conditions that respond to the relaxation response. There are likely others, but he clearly proved efficacy in treating angina pectoris, cardiac arrhythmias, allergic skin reactions, anxiety, mild to moderate depression, bronchial asthma, herpes simplex, cough, constipation, diabetes mellitus, duodenal ulcers, dizziness, fatigue, hypertension, infertility, insomnia, nausea and vomiting during pregnancy, nervousness, postoperative swelling, premenstrual syndrome, rheumatoid arthritis, side effects of cancer, side effects of AIDS, and all forms of pain—backaches, headaches, abdominal pain, muscle pain, joint aches, postoperative pain, and neck, arm, and leg pain.

In his 1975 book *The Relaxation Response*, Benson announced that he had discovered a counterbalance to the fight-or-flight response Cannon had described decades earlier. Just as the body has a natural survival mechanism built in to help you run away from a wild animal, the body also has an inducible, physiological state of quietude, which allows the body to repair damage done by the fight-or-flight response.

After his book hit the *New York Times* bestseller list, Benson got a lot of media attention and was admonished by his peers because "physicians at Harvard do not write popular books." His colleagues continued to critique him, claiming that the relaxation response was merely a placebo effect. Because patients believed it would lower their blood pressure, it did. In other words, it was belief that made the technique effective, not the actual technique.

Because, at the time, he had as much disdain for the placebo effect as his colleagues did, Benson worked diligently to prove that the relaxation response was a distinct physiological state. What he found was that the relaxation response worked more than a placebo comparison; however, even though his technique was more effective than placebo, the placebo arm of the study still worked 50 to 90 percent of the time. Benson realized that the placebo effect was not something to be scoffed at but rather something to harness. He proposed renaming the placebo effect "remembered wellness" and suggested that it was a useful counterpart to the verifiable physiological state those eliciting the relaxation response could induce.

Benson's continued research found that regular elicitation of the relaxation response could prevent and compensate for the damaging effects of stress on the body, warding off disease and sometimes treating it. Benson wanted to know if the same response could be elicited in other activities besides meditation, so he kept up his research and found four essential components that could reliably elicit the relaxation response: 1) a quiet environment; 2) a mental device, such as a repeated phrase, word, sound, or prayer; 3) a passive, nonjudgmental attitude; and 4) a comfortable position.

Later, he discovered that only the mental device and passive attitude were necessary. A runner with a mantra and a passive attitude could be jogging down a busy street and elicit a relaxation response. The same was true for those doing yoga or qigong, walking, swimming, knitting, rowing, sitting, standing, dancing, making art, or singing. As he continued a lifetime of research, Benson found that the majority of medical problems were either caused by or exacerbated by the chronic effects of the stress response on the body. Other studies showed that from 60 to 90 percent of doctor visits could be attributed to the stress response.[1,2]

Intuitively, we know this, and when we're stressed out, we crave relaxation. But too often, we go about it the wrong way, seeking out unhealthy forms of stress relief like alcohol, tobacco, and illegal drugs, which only exacerbate the problem. There are, however, healthy ways to elicit the relaxation response—such as meditation—that are the best medicine we can take for treatment of life's stresses.

To test the effectiveness of elicitation of the relaxation response on the body, Benson invented a way to teach patients how to elicit this response in a way that wasn't as woo-woo as Transcendental Meditation or as spiritual as prayer.

How to Elicit the Relaxation Response

(from Herbert Benson's *The Relaxation Response*)

1. Pick a focus word, short phrase, or prayer that is firmly rooted in your belief system, such as "one," "peace," "The Lord is my shepherd," "Hail Mary, full of grace," "Shalom," or "Om."

2. Sit quietly in a comfortable position.

3. Close your eyes.

4. Relax your muscles, progressing from your feet to your calves, thighs, abdomen, shoulders, head, and neck.

5. Breathe slowly and naturally, and as you do, say your focus word, sound, phrase, or prayer silently to yourself as you exhale.

6. Assume a passive attitude. Don't worry about how well you're doing. When other thoughts come to mind, simply say to yourself, "Oh, well," and gently return to your repetition.

7. Continue for 10 to 20 minutes.

8. Do not stand immediately. Continue sitting quietly for a minute or so, allowing other thoughts to return. Then open your eyes and sit for another minute before rising.

9. Practice the technique once or twice daily. Good times to do so are before breakfast and before dinner.[3]

This technique was found to be highly effective for eliciting the relaxation response and improving health. But in his latest book, *Timeless Healing: The Power and Biology of Belief*, Benson provides updated information on how to elicit the relaxation response. Essentially, this is all you need:

A Simplified Way to Elicit the Relaxation Response

- Repetition of a word, sound, phrase, prayer, or muscular activity.

- Passively disregarding everyday thoughts that inevitably come to mind and returning to your repetition.

This can be done while exercising, making art, dancing, cooking, shopping, driving . . . whatever.

Psychoneuroimmunology

Benson's research launched the mind-body connection into mass consciousness, but it was neuroscientist, pharmacologist, and researcher Candace Pert, Ph.D., who really deserves the credit for much of our scientific understanding of what we now call "the mind-body connection." Deemed "The Mother of Psychoneuroimmunology," she authored over 250 research papers that revolutionized our understanding about how our thoughts, beliefs, and feelings translate into the "molecules of emotion" that tie the mind, consciousness, and emotions to the physical body. She writes, "My argument is that the three classic areas of neuroscience, endocrinology, and immunology, with their various organs—the brain (which is the key organ that the neuroscientists study), the glands, and the immune system (consisting of the spleen, the bone marrow, the lymph nodes, and of course the cells circulating throughout the body)—that these three areas are actually joined to each other in a bidirectional network of communication and that the information 'carriers' are the neuropeptides." As she describes in her best-selling book *The Molecules of Emotion: The Science Behind Mind-Body Medicine*, it is these neuropeptide hormones that make up the biochemical soup of both disease and healing, depending on what concoction arises.

This was a revolutionary, controversial, and disruptive discovery at a time when reductionist medicine was at its peak, but given her credentials, it was hard for the establishment to write off this accomplished, scientifically rigorous John Hopkins graduate. The field of psychoneuroimmunology is now an established scientific discipline, offering a grounded link between the spiritual realm of consciousness and the scientific realms of neuroscience and medicine, due in large part to Pert's contributions to the field.

Meditation

You don't have to follow Benson's prescription for eliciting the relaxation response. Other forms of meditation offer great health benefits that have been well documented. All forms of meditation, to some degree, activate the parasympathetic nervous system, decrease stress-related cortisol, reduce respiration and heart rate, reduce the metabolic rate, increase blood flow in the brain, strengthen the immune system, lead to a state of relaxation, and activate the neural changes that lead to bliss brain.[4]

Meditation also reduces pain, work stress, anxiety, and depression, promotes cardiovascular health, improves cognitive function, lowers blood pressure, reduces alcohol abuse, improves longevity, promotes healthy weight, reduces tension headaches, relieves asthma, controls blood sugar in diabetic patients, alleviates PMS, reduces chronic pain, improves immune function, and raises quality of life.[5]

Keep in mind that meditation is a broad umbrella that covers a wide variety of ways to relax your nervous system, leading to altered states of consciousness, and not all meditations are created equal! Every spiritual tradition has its own forms of meditation, and there are many secular forms of meditation as well. One of my spiritual mentors defines meditation as "being aware that you're aware." In other words, if you're not absorbed in "selfing," thinking you are your thoughts, then you become the witness of your thoughts, as well as everything else that is happening around you. This state of consciousness, which some spiritual teachers call "witness consciousness," can become stabilized with some practice, and at that point, everything becomes a meditation. But staying permanently in witness consciousness can also lead to detachment and disembodiment, which is not ultimately a healing practice. Embodiment is necessary for healing the body. In order to heal the body, your body needs your blessing, your presence, and the light of your awareness bathing every cell with the rapturous radiance of love.

Some meditation practices, the cooling practices, happen in the lotus position, in stillness on a pillow, while other meditation practices, the warming practices, happen through movement, singing, and merging with the divine in nature with eyes wide open. Some use focus techniques like Benson's TM mantra, a candle flame, the sound of a singing bowl, or the breath. Others invite you to follow sensations in the body, emotions in the body, or spontaneous or positional movements of the body (such as qigong, yoga asanas, or dance.) Anything that quiets the DMN, relaxes the mental chatter, and puts you in touch with your essence, the One, the energy of consciousness, the earth, or the frequency of a particular deity can do the job of turning off stress responses in the body and activating the relaxation response. But if you're focusing on transcendent practices, true healing always requires coming back into the body.

Keep in mind that many traditional meditation practices lack balance between sacred masculine and sacred feminine energies. The cooling, detached masculine practices prioritize transcending this reality, going beyond the body, getting out of yourself, and merging your consciousness with silence, emptiness, or what some call "the void." The warming, heart-opening feminine practices focus on embodiment, feeling and moving with your emotions, opening the heart to feel love and compassion for all of your parts and all beings, feeling your passion for life, justice, and sacred activism, and really grounding in form and matter. Whether you're male or female, both kinds of practices can benefit your consciousness and your health. People who identify as male may find transcendent practices more natural, while those who identify as female may find embodiment practices to be more resonant—but both are necessary to awaken in your spiritual development and optimize your health.

However you go about it, meditation is an effective antidote to chronic repetitive stress responses and a powerful healing practice that has many other transformational benefits. Meditation is one of the most health-inducing behaviors you can engage in, not just for your spiritual development, but also for your emotional health, your mental health, your creativity, your intuition, your embodied sexuality, and your physical health. It's the *being* that balances the out-of-control *doing* of our society's cultural programming. If you're not used to doing nothing, being may feel like a supreme waste of time. But trust me when I say it's not. It's one of the best uses of your time you can possibly prioritize, especially if you're on a healing journey.

Creating Sacred Space

If you've never meditated before, you might enjoy designating a sacred space where it feels good to settle yourself for meditation practice. I create altars in my home so it feels like a very personal temple space, where I collect special objects I've gathered from sacred sites all over the world—holy water from Lourdes, a wrought-iron heart fitted into an iron box that I found in Big Sur, a piece of rose quartz a friend gave me, a condor feather, a small statue a patient gave me, a painting a dear friend made, a framed photo, a cup of sand from the River Jordan, a crucifix with *milagros* from the Santuario de Chimayó, some *palo santo* from Peru, a pinecone from my backyard, a candle, some incense, and a bowl of fresh gardenias. My altars are living, breathing prayers, so I change them often and set different intentions for different altars. All you need to start your own temple is an empty closet or a corner in your bedroom where you can gather meaningful objects and arrange them in a way that feels right to you. I also love meditating out in nature, under a tree, on the beach, by the river, or on top of a mountain. Beauty can be a potent gateway to the rapture of the divine in all things.

How to Meditate

If you're new to meditation, you may find it helpful to start with guided meditations and visualizations, such as the ones I've recorded in my *Ignite Your Inner Pilot Light Meditations* mp3 (LissaRankin.com). Sometimes it's easier to listen to someone else's guiding voice than to face the chatter that tends to show up the minute your eyes are closed and the room is silent. If my meditations aren't your cup o'tea, try the scientifically sculpted "eco-meditation" created by EFT teacher Dawson Church, Ph.D. (ecomeditation.com). Or try Belleruth Naparstek's extensive library of meditations that are specific to various physical and mental health conditions (HealthJourneys.com). If healing trauma and becoming more intimate with and healing all parts of yourself is a priority for you, I highly recommend the Internal Family Systems (IFS) guided meditations *Meditations for Self* created by Richard Schwartz, Ph.D. (ifs-institute.com). If what you're seeking is altered states of consciousness through neuroscience, try the Monroe Institute's Hemi-Sync meditations, which create a focused, whole-brain state known as hemispheric synchronization, where the left and right hemispheres are working together in a state of coherence (monroeinstitute.org). Tune in to your inner knowing and feel into which guided meditation might be the right place to start.

If you feel ready for silence, prepare to discover what happens in your mind when it's not stimulated. This can be surprising at first. You may feel all kinds of emotions that get suppressed by excessive busyness, you may notice that your thoughts are racing, or you may become aware of discomfort in your body that you've been ignoring. Don't judge what happens. Remember, this is about being, so just be with what is—and breathe.

Once you find a comfortable position, close your eyes to minimize visual distractions, and try focusing on your breath as you inhale and exhale. Buddhist meditation teacher Jack Kornfield suggests that if you notice yourself remembering, planning, or fantasizing, refrain from judging yourself, but do call it out: "Hello, remembering." "Hello, planning." "Hello, fantasizing." Welcome whatever arises, and don't demonize your emotions or your thoughts.

Just be with them and send them your care and attention. Then return to the present moment, focusing on your breath. The minute you notice your thoughts starting to wander, come back to your breath. To circumvent distracting images that may appear in your mind, you may also try scanning your body for any parts that don't feel relaxed and visualizing your breath going to those tense spots. Imagine your breath as golden light flowing to the tense places and filling them with relaxation. Relax your back, your shoulders, your belly, your facial muscles. Try tensing and releasing each muscle, starting at your forehead and moving down your body all the way to your toes.

If your only experience in meditation is to pop out of your body, you might stretch yourself by trying deep soul embodiment practices, which help to bring the soul all the way into the body. Start with a HeartMath practice, locating your awareness in your heart and breathing in and out through your heart, as if your heart were lungs, allowing yourself to simultaneously feel something you're sincerely and utterly grateful for. Breathe that gratitude in and out of your heart until you feel your heart open.

Then add on this yoga practice, feeling the blossoming of the light in your heart as the light expands as wide as your torso. Let that light fill your torso and drop through your body, like a column of light coming out of your bottom, coursing through the soil and into the bedrock, and landing at the core of the earth as if it were plugging into the earth's energetic heart. Allow anything that no longer serves you to release down that grounding cord, into the earth's center, where it can get composted by the Earth Mother. You can also visualize this grounding energy of the earth's core coursing up through your body and filling you with healing earth energy. Then imagine cosmic light energy coming through the top of your head, bringing with it any wisdom, insight, intuition, or healing that may be available. Now let this heavenly light expand in your head, and drop another column of light all the way down your body, meeting the earth energy in the center of your heart. Breathe in and out through your heart. Then let this light move up and down the core of your body as one. Breathe light down into the earth with the exhale, imagining the light sinking into the earth's crust, then breathe light from beneath the earth all the way up out through the top of your head with the inhale, squeezing your core muscles as you breathe. Squeeze and breathe as you shoot this light out through the top of your head. Now bring it back down into the earth with the exhale. Keep cycling this energy with your breath, seeing yourself as the light of breath as it moves up and down through your core, clearing blocks and healing the body as it moves in you. Stay in the feeling of gratitude if you can. Feel how lucky you are to be a soul in form, incarnated in this beautiful body of yours.

Over time, as you become intimate with all the multiplicity of parts in you—including the thoughts, sensations, and emotions those parts may generate—your parts are likely to relax, calm down, and give you more space so you can begin to experience more spaciousness with an empty mind, open heart, and blissed-out brain. But don't get discouraged if this takes time. Meditation is like training a puppy. You just keep practicing your discipline, and over time, it gets easier. Given enough time, it's likely to become your favorite part of the day.

If sitting meditation doesn't do it for you, and especially if you identify more with feminine energies, try a somatic meditation and movement practice I learned from Kashmir Shaivism Tantra teacher Michaela Boehm, author of *The Wild Woman's Way*. Start on hands and knees on a yoga mat, and choose a playlist of evocative music that moves you. Now simply let your body spontaneously move however it wants to move. Stay on your mat. This isn't a full-on dance practice, though if that happens, go for it. The intention is to just stay with whatever fluid movement arises as your body tunes in to the music and feels into what feels pleasurable in your body in the moment. Over time, this can be a very powerful practice that helps you calm your nervous system, process your emotions, awaken sensation and sexual energy, release trauma from the body, unite mind and body, create body responsiveness, and open you up to the wise guidance of bodily wisdom.

If you still find yourself resisting, it may be because you have a lot of unhealed trauma in your system, and the hurt parts are scared you'll get too close to the intense feelings they carry. The parts that resist may be trying to make sure you don't get taken out by too many painful emotions, preventing you from showing up for life's responsibilities. If this is the case, don't force yourself. Your protective parts are there for a reason. Find a good therapist, and get the help you deserve.

Other Ways to Elicit the Relaxation Response

It's not just meditation that shuts off the stress response and calms the body. As we've learned, expressing yourself creatively, achieving sexual release, being with people you love, spending time with your spiritual community, doing work that feeds your soul, and other relaxing activities such as laughing, playing with pets, journaling, praying, napping, doing yoga or tai chi, getting a massage, reading, singing, playing a musical instrument, gardening, cooking, going for a walk, taking a hot bath, and enjoying nature may also activate your parasympathetic nervous system and allow the body to return to a state of rest so it can go about the business of self-repair.

This is vital for every single one of us, not just as treatment for illness but for prevention of it and extension of our lives. According to the American Psychiatric Association's 2017 "Stress in America" survey, three out of four Americans reported experiencing at least one stress symptom in the last month, including lying awake at night, feeling nervous or anxious, or experiencing fatigue due to stress.[6] While stress can be hard to avoid, the relaxation response can serve as a counterbalancing medicinal factor.

Can't quit your stressful job? Not ready to leave your unhappy marriage? Haven't found the love of your life yet? Not interested in going to church? That's okay. I'm not suggesting you have to do everything I've covered in this book in order to be optimally healthy. But I am suggesting that if you're exposed to stressors you either can't change or aren't ready to change, you must prioritize activities that induce the relaxation response as a way to counterbalance the stresses in your life. Part of how meditation helps you spend more time in the relaxation response is by developing your consciousness to the point that even the seemingly stressful or painful events that are a natural part of being human can be experienced fully, felt and expressed passionately, integrated into the body, and then moved as vital energy through your body without precipitating disease. In other words, you might not need to make big life shifts in order to shift your nervous system into relaxation responses a greater percentage of the time. Sometimes what works best is shifting your consciousness, such that even life's challenges become an opportunity for gratitude and growth. This is not meant to be a "spiritual bypass" that grooms you to tolerate abuse in the name of showing how "conscious" you are; in fact, healing yourself might require you to initiate conflict and make some tough changes. This might also require you to feel emotional pain, which you can handle more easily with the right kind of meditation practice, one that helps you host your painful feelings without trying to transcend them.

A regular meditation practice allows us to more easily host whatever arises in our human experience, allowing these waves of emotion to move through us so we can do what we can to heal the pain from the root, without bypassing it. In this way, if you're grounded in a daily meditation practice and facing the circumstances of your life with an awakening consciousness, then if big, potentially painful changes need to happen in your day-to-day life, you'll find the strength to lovingly but firmly lean into the conflict and be with the pain rather than resisting it. The guidance you'll tune in to inside yourself will then come from embodied intuition. In this way, your nervous system will rest in the peace of the parasympathetic response more and more, and this prepares the foundation for the possibility of radical remission.

Rx for Self-Healing

Now that I've pointed out how the stress responses that originate in your mind and impact your nervous system damage your body, you might be expecting me to dole out a specific prescription for exactly how you can alleviate loneliness, find love, enjoy better sex, reduce work stress, earn more, be more creative, feel happier, deepen your spiritual development, and relax the body. After all, I'm a doctor. We write prescriptions, right?

Although we all crave quick fixes and long to believe that some expert finally has the one secret solution to all our problems, the truth is that you'd probably be annoyed if I tried to write your prescription for you. Any efforts on my part to do so, even those based on cold, hard science, would likely come across as trite. Just picture it.

If you don't believe you can get well, switch out your negative beliefs for positive ones. If you're lonely, join a club, sign up for online dating, and find the right spiritual community. If you're stressed at work, quit and find a better job. If you feel creatively thwarted, start creating. If you're broke, earn more. If you're a pessimist, become an optimist. If you're unhappy, get happier. If you feel stressed, relax.

Easy for me to say.

Whether you're trying to recover from a health condition or prevent disease until you die of old age, the process is the same. In Part Three of this book, I'm going to teach you the six steps to healing yourself so you can write your own Prescription. (Don't worry! No medical-school education required.)

Remember, I'm not suggesting you ditch your doctor or avoid the hospital. If your intuitive guidance includes conventional medicine as part of your self-healing Prescription, *please* take advantage of all the miracles modern medical technology has added to the medicine bag! Nothing irritates me more than when people misinterpret what I'm teaching and falsely conclude that I'm recommending they turn their backs on modern medicine. I wouldn't recommend skipping that surgery when you have appendicitis or not taking that antibiotic when you have a severe infection. And if you're in a car accident and your body breaks from the sheer brute force of an automobile crushing you, or if you're having a heart attack or stroke, get thee to a Level I Trauma Center STAT! Trauma care is what modern medicine does best. Medical technology can save your life in acute medical emergency situations and buy you time if you get help right away.

While writing your Prescription will certainly increase your body's ability to repair itself when something does go wrong, I'd never want you to risk your life by delaying treatment if you're suffering from a potentially life- or limb-threatening disease. I want to make it clear that what I'll be teaching you in Part Three works best as a path for healing: for chronic illness or disability; as part of a holistic cancer regimen that might also include conventional medical treatment; as an adjunct to the rehabilitation process for people who have just had medical interventions in acute emergencies like a heart attack, stroke, or automobile accident; as treatment for those who have been diagnosed with mental illness; or as preventive medicine for those aiming to extend their life expectancy with a high quality of life.

Beyond the scope of this book, but bearing mention for those looking to achieve optimal health, are holistic and preventive health tips your conventional doctor might not bring up. While the treatment plan you're about to create is primarily aimed at healing your mental, emotional, and spiritual health, you'll also need to prioritize engaging in what we consider traditional healthy behaviors, such as using food as medicine, exercising daily, getting enough sleep, avoiding toxic exposures, balancing your hormones, and addressing the kinds of issues functional medicine doctors address well. You can work yourself silly shifting your beliefs, healing your trauma, alleviating loneliness, eliminating work and financial stress, and treating your depression and anxiety, but if you're still drinking, smoking, and eating highly processed microwavable dinners, that just ain't gonna cut it. Not only does your mind need the right nutrition for healthy brain activity, the endorphins of regular exercise, and the rest of a good night's sleep, but your body also needs to be nourished and protected from the hazards of an increasingly chemicalized environment.

When patients on a mission to heal themselves from a "chronic" or "incurable" illness seek my guidance, I always recommend adding green juice as a daily supplement, eating as many raw foods (go veggies!) as you can, limiting meat or choosing animal products wisely, eliminating processed foods, adding superfoods like chlorella, spirulina, seaweed, and wheatgrass to their diets, and eliminating or at least cutting back on white sugar, gluten, caffeine, alcohol, tobacco, and illegal drugs. I personally do a 21-day raw foods/green juice detox cleanse once or twice as year as preventive medicine.

While some "health-conscious" people use raw foods and cleansing as a cover for eating disorders, used in a wise and psychologically healthy manner, such nutrient-rich, food-as-medicine cleanses can be a purifying reset for the body, mind, and spirit.

I also recommend optimizing the biochemistry of the body by visiting a conscious, open-minded functional medicine or integrative medicine doctor familiar with balancing and optimizing the body's hormones and neurotransmitters and using natural substances to boost the immune system and foster the body's natural healing powers. Many of our Whole Health Medicine Institute graduates, who have been trained in a variety of psychospiritual healing methods, including the Six Steps to Healing Yourself, also have integrative or functional medicine practices. (Find practitioners near you at WholeHealthMedicineInstitute.com.)

It's also crucial to be cognizant of the environment in which you live. Are you living a "green" life? Are you being exposed to harmful chemicals in plastics, pesticides, toxic household chemicals, heavy metals, mold, or asbestos? The World Health Organization (WHO) reports that 24 percent of global disease is caused by environmental exposures that could be averted. They estimate that more than 33 percent of diseases in children under the age of five are caused by environmental exposures and posit that addressing environmental issues could save as many as 4 million lives a year in children alone, mostly in developing countries.[7]

Clearly, you can do everything "right" when it comes to nurturing your mental, emotional, and spiritual health, but if your body is full of poison, either from your diet, what you drink, or your environment, a healthy nervous system just won't counteract the damage you're inflicting upon your vulnerable body.

Others address these issues in more detail, and this will not be the primary focus of what we'll address in Part Three, though I will trust that you'll do your homework and get expert help in order to make any additions necessary to address the external causes of poor health that might be impacting you. What I'll focus on is the elephant in the room that most doctors and health, diet, and fitness folks ignore: mental, emotional, and spiritual healing as part of any complete treatment plan. Using a six-step process for how to listen to your body, diagnose the root of what might be causing or exacerbating your illness, and create a treatment plan for yourself aimed at reducing stress responses and eliciting relaxation responses so the body can be returned to its natural capacity for self-healing, you'll become your own doctor and healer. Ready, set, heal!

PART THREE

THE SIX STEPS TO HEALING YOURSELF

CHAPTER 9

THE SIX STEPS TO HEALING YOURSELF

It's supposed to be a professional secret, but I'll tell you anyway. We doctors do nothing. We only help and encourage the doctor within.

— ALBERT SCHWEITZER, M.D.

If you decide you're ready to embark upon the Six Steps to Healing Yourself, you'll be venturing on a journey of transformation that is guaranteed to change your life. You don't have to wait until your body starts yelling with some life-threatening illness to make life changes that will increase your likelihood of being a health outlier. You don't even have to have a physical illness to benefit from the Six Steps, since this process works to help you transform whatever in your life may need healing.

In this section, I'm going to teach you a scientifically grounded process I used with my patients back when I was still practicing medicine. This process is now the foundation of the curriculum of the Whole Health Medicine Institute, which many physicians, therapists, and healers around the world are using with patients. I have honed and modified these six steps since the first edition of this book, so you will benefit from nearly a decade of experience working with these transformational healing steps. These six steps have not yet been prospectively studied to scientifically prove that they impact disease outcomes, but each step is grounded in the scientific research I've shared with you in Part One and Part Two of this book. Although any scientist knows that anecdotes do not make good

science, what I can say is that the anecdotes we've been privy to hear from the doctors and patients who have applied the methods in this book suggest that, at least for some people, making these changes in your life can be very healing, and at times, radically curative, even when you've been told cure is impossible.

Before we get started, I want to make one final distinction. Throughout this book, I've used the words *healing* and *curing* interchangeably. When we talk about healing a fracture, we usually mean curing a fracture (the broken bone grows back together). In this instance, they mean the same thing. But the etymology of the word "heal" is the Old English hælan, which translates as "to make whole." To be cured means to be free of disease or symptoms. So there's actually a difference between healing and curing. It's possible to be healed but not cured, and it's possible to be cured but not healed. Ideally, healing and curing happen together, but this isn't always the case.

So what does it mean to be healed? When you are healed, wholeness is restored at a level that transcends the body but can also include the body. Whether or not your illness resolves, healing is possible, as anyone who has witnessed a beautiful death can verify. When you're dealing with an illness, being sick can be an opportunity for spiritual awakening, and when you awaken your consciousness, grounding and embodying your spiritual essence fully into every cell of the body, you return to your natural state of wholeness. This state of wholeness puts the mind and body in an optimally relaxed state so the self-repair mechanisms of the body can best do their job and life force can course through you, bringing with it the conditions that help the body restore optimal function.

If that's the case, why doesn't everyone who works the Six Steps faithfully wind up cured? Why does one person experience radical remission and another doesn't? The truth is that nobody knows the answer to this question. Some believe that all illness is the result of disordered thinking, that even if your conscious mind believes you can get well, you'll be sabotaged if your subconscious mind disagrees with you. Some believe that disease is the result of blocked energy in the "biofield," with energetic interference preceding the physical manifestation of disease, and if the biofield stays blocked, no intervention that doesn't involve clearing this block will lead to the desired outcome. Others believe that illness results from harmful behaviors committed in past lives, which must be atoned for in this one—that it's karma that much be expiated. Still others cite divine destiny or believe that your soul chooses to experience certain hardships in a body in order learn lessons here in "earth school" as a way to develop one's consciousness over lifetimes. Some believe that unavoidable tragedies simply happen at random; they claim that our psychological or spiritual attempts to make meaning out of our suffering are just a cover for our discomfort with the uncertainty of an uncontrollable universe and that there's simply no way to avoid having bad things happen to good people.

I'm not here to discuss theology or spout off about things I don't fully understand, but I also don't want to skirt the issue altogether. So what's my point of view? Why are some cured when they heal and others aren't? All I can say is this: when my patients have been ready and willing to engage in deep inquiry regarding psycho-spiritual trauma-healing work, stayed open to lifestyle modifications aimed at living a more aligned Inner Pilot Light-led life, and remained willing to sacrifice comfort, certainty, and security in favor of authenticity, self-compassion, relational and spiritual healing, and a commitment to life purpose, seemingly miraculous feats of physical self-repair have sometimes happened. *The same thing could happen to you.*

If you're prepared to embark upon this journey and the time is now, I encourage you to seek support from someone you trust, with whom you can share what might come up for you. Ideally this will be someone trained and experienced in the process of helping people navigate emotional issues and traumas when they arise, such as a licensed therapist, mental health counselor, psychiatrist, spiritual advisor, or graduate of the Whole Health Medicine Institute (Whole HealthMedicineInstitute.com), where health-care providers are trained to help you navigate the six self-healing steps outlined in this book. If healing trauma winds up being a core piece of your healing work, please seek out someone experienced in the cutting-edge trauma therapies, such as Advanced Integrative Therapy (AIT), Internal Family Systems (IFS), Somatic Experiencing (SE), or Emotional Freedom

Techniques (EFT), among others. You can find practitioners trained in these advanced trauma healing modalities on websites dedicated to each modality. The paradox of healing is that your body can heal itself, but you can't do it alone. Translating transformational work into a self-help book misses a key element of healing—the person or people who love you unconditionally, without judgment or agenda, who hold the space for wounds to heal and your body to heal itself. Please don't deprive yourself of the gift of such a healing presence if you are in a position to find one.

I want to acknowledge that this way of approaching adversity as an opportunity for awakening is not for everyone. One of the most common questions people ask me is, "How can I make my [mother/father/spouse/patient/client] open up to what you teach in *Mind Over Medicine*?" My answer is that you are always free to offer a gentle invitation to anyone who you think might benefit from these insights, revelations, and healing practices. But keep in mind that everyone is entitled to his or her own journey. You've heard that you can lead a horse to water but you can't make him drink. Some people are too rigid in their beliefs, anchored in scientific materialism, and shut down from unhealed trauma to even consider approaching illness in this way. And that is their right. Everyone is entitled to navigate illness the way they choose to do so. There is no need to convert anyone or demonize anyone if they choose to turn away from the opportunity for transformation that this book offers. Should you find yourself frustrated because some people are not open to this way of healing, prioritize healing the parts of you that are understandably scared of losing someone you love or watching them suffer, while also healing the parts of yourself that think you have any business controlling someone else's healing journey. A healing journey like the one this book invites is a uniquely individual experience, a rabbit hole of its own, and it takes gumption, resilience, and a whole lot of loving support from yourself and from those who will nurture you through this process. If you or someone you love is not up for this, please be gentle, patient, and compassionate.

If, however, you feel ready, let's get started. You have everything to gain as you reclaim who you really are, align with your truth, and make your body ripe for miracles. Whether or not you cure your body, I guarantee your life will improve if you follow the steps I'm about to teach you. I believe in you, so please . . . come.

The Six Steps as a Learning Process

As is often the case with works in progress, The Six Steps to Healing Yourself have evolved as I've learned from experience. When I was talking to Richard Schwartz about how the Internal Family Systems (IFS) model came to be, he told me that developing the IFS model has required him to be willing to be wrong dozens of times in the thirty years he has spent creating it. Since the first edition of *Mind Over Medicine*, I've learned so much and proven myself wrong time and again. Any good scientist needs to be willing to assert a hypothesis, test the hypothesis, and then collect evidence that either proves or disproves the hypothesis without attachment to whether the hypothesis is right or wrong. When the number one priority is the quest for truth, rather than a dogmatic agenda aimed at being right, the truth will continue to reveal itself over time.

I was originally trying to take a method I'd used to treat people one on one and scale it to teach groups of hundreds. The attempt made the blind spots glaringly obvious. Part of what induced the new, revised Six Steps in this edition was a rising awareness that many people who are sick are sincerely desperate to get well on a conscious level. But on a deeper unconscious level, many people with chronic or life-threatening illnesses are getting deep core needs met by being sick. Sometimes terms like "secondary gain" are used to describe this, but such language can sound shaming or suggest intentional manipulation to many clients, so I prefer to use other language. Let's say that some people have hurt parts or protective parts of their personality that at a subconscious level think the illness is necessary in order to get essential needs met, needs like love, attention, security, approval, or money. Illness may give someone a valid, socially acceptable excuse to stop over-caregiving for others, get out of responsibilities they don't want to fulfill, or avoid risking failure by trying to realize a dream. Such impulses usually live way down in someone's blind spot, so they're unconscious but powerful energetic blocks that can impede cure. While these people will *say* they want to get well—and consciously they do—the mind operates from the subconscious mind 95 percent of the time. So if 5 percent of your mind wants to get well but 95 percent of your mind doesn't, the force of your co-creative power goes toward creating illness, not wellness. In other words, you're successful at manifesting what you want, only you're manifesting from the unconscious mind, not the conscious mind. The work of healing requires bringing the conscious and unconscious mind together with what I call your Inner Pilot Light. Healing lies in this reunion of wholeness.

Let me give you a few examples. One man who worked the six steps suddenly realized he didn't want to give up his disability check and go back to a soul-sucking job, but he didn't know how else to provide for the family and wasn't interested in being creative about how else he could make money. A woman realized that cancer was serving a purpose to make her prioritize her own needs instead of caregiving a sick parent, but she wasn't willing to endure the guilt of abandoning her father in a state of need, so it was easier to stay sick than to assert herself and say no to her father and other family members. One man suddenly saw how illness was a good excuse to avoid toxic family gatherings. A woman realized that her illness helped her get out of housework and child care duties and also gave her a good reason for not writing the book she'd always dreamed of writing. In other words, their illnessses were *protecting* them, even while also creating suffering and potentially putting their lives at stake. Energetically, because you have two opposing forces fighting each other, you put one foot on the gas and one foot on the brakes. But those pedals might not be equal. If 5 percent is pushing the gas pedal, but 95 percent is on the brakes, the stuck densities in the body that can cause illness are unlikely to move.

People often feel ashamed when they realize this, but there is no shame in finally facing what has been true in the subconscious and is now being made conscious in the light of awareness. By shining the light of consciousness—and the unconditional love of your Inner Pilot Light—upon this block, you take back the reins and reclaim your power consciously. Becoming aware of your blocks and clearing them allows you to quit fighting yourself. If you really want to optimize outcomes, you'll need to address these blocks and clear them so that if cure is in the cards for your soul's journey, it can become possible.

To address this issue, I've adjusted the original Six Steps as follows: I've added a step about dealing with the inevitable fear and resistance that arises, and clearing those blocks. I also moved the order of some of the steps and collapsed two steps into one.

So . . . to review:

The New Six Steps to Healing Yourself

Step One: Believe that healing is possible. In the co-creative process, you don't control the outcome, but you do get to cast your vote! If you believe you're incurable, terminal, or chronically ill, that's the vote you're casting. If, however, you're willing to question your beliefs and open yourself to the possibility that healing could happen and cure might be in the cards for you, you open a portal of possibility. Once you've removed the anchored belief that cure is not possible, you make yourself available to become a "health outlier," someone who has the potential to have a better-than-expected outcome. Savoring the possibility of cure can give you an inner experience of elevated emotions evoked by the possibility of a miraculous outcome. How would that feel, to be free of this condition that causes you to suffer? Can you give yourself that experience as a potential outcome and fully relish in your imagination how that would feel? If you don't believe it's possible that you might heal, you may need to be proactive about shifting your beliefs with the practices you will learn in this chapter to help you let go of limiting beliefs and replace them with health-inducing ones. It's fine to acknowledge the uncertainty that accompanies any healing journey and allow yourself to feel the feelings that might come with uncertainty—fear, grief, disappointment, frustration, despair. But also remember that when you don't know what the future holds, *anything is possible,* even a miracle. Can you let yourself dance with the unknown? Go ahead and educate yourself about the statistics of your prognosis if it calms the part that wants to know and helps you manage your expectations and assess your situation with a realistic lens. But keep in mind that you are not a statistic. You are a unique individual who has an unknown and unknowable future. This is not about entering a state of false hope or denial. It's about removing blocks to the doorway of healing and then walking all the way through that doorway into grounded hope.

Step Two: Connect and surrender to your Inner Pilot Light, letting your inner knowing guide your healing journey. Step Two is about developing the internal support and guidance you'll need to navigate your journey to healing. Once you allow yourself to believe that healing is possible for you, the next step is surrendering your attachment to outcomes. This is no small feat when you're suffering and desperate for relief. How do you let go of the desire for cure when your very life may be at stake? Some people may choose to surrender to a higher power outside themselves—God, Buddha, Allah, Jesus, an archangel, a guide, or a guru. Others may prefer to surrender to the Divine healer within, which I call your "Inner Pilot Light." However you access it, solidifying your connection to this higher power and accessing it inside your own being is the key to your healing. Of course you want to be healed, but the heaviness of that longing can keep you stuck in the frequency of understandably desperate grasping. Don't try to suppress your desire for healing. Let yourself be *on fire with* your desire for healing, then cast the burden of this intense desire over to whatever spiritual Source you trust and ask for help navigating your healing journey. Trust that if right action is required, you will be guided and shown what to do. Allow yourself to be bathed in gratitude for all the help that will come to support you emotionally, physically, and spiritually as you acknowledge the jnterconnected web of life by connecting to your Inner Pilot Light. Make the humble action of admitting that you can't do this alone, that you will need guidance from the healing energy that courses through this web. Once you let go of thinking you can control this process, intuition, signs and synchronicities, body wisdom, and whatever else you will need to navigate this path will come your way. Once you are connected to this web of life with your act of surrender, you can no longer remain separate from it and it can rise to support your journey. Fill yourself with the knowing that help is here. This step is a call to action, an opening to the guidance that can be received, interpreted, discerned, and followed via your Inner Pilot Light. The rational mind can be helpful to analyze treatment options and other choices you'll need to make, but nothing beats your Inner Pilot Light for shining the clarity of your inner knowing on the aligned path.

Step Three: Surround yourself with healing support. While connecting to your Inner Pilot Light gives you the internal support you'll need, you'll also need external support in the form of a healing team. As much as some self-help books like to suggest that healing can be a solitary journey, optimal healing does not usually arise from the consciousness of the rugged individualist. Perhaps part of the healing process is intended to restore your place of belonging in the tribe. If you believe you have to do everything yourself and you can't dare to rely on anyone else's love and support, that's a recipe for illness. No wonder your body would feel the need to force you to receive care! Even if you're an introvert or a monk, you'll need the right kind of support. Keep in mind that great support might come from your loved ones, but you will likely also need experts, whether they are doctors, therapists, CAM providers, or healers. Discerning carefully who has a seat at your "Healing Round Table" could save your life. Let your Inner Pilot Light be the one who chooses who supports you.

Step Four: Diagnose the root cause of your illness. The Whole Health Cairn wellness model is the foundation of this step. The Whole Health Cairn is designed to give you a framework for taking inventory of the facets of a balanced life, so you can intuit where you are living in alignment with your truth and following your heart—and where you're not. Pay close attention to the insights that arise as you contemplate the health of your relationships, your work, your creative life, your sexuality, your relationship to spirituality and your Inner Pilot Light, your relationship to scarcity or abundance, your living environment, your mental health, and how you treat your body physically with traditionally healthy behaviors. Healing is the natural state of the human body, so when healing stops and disease takes over, it's important to identify what led to an interruption of the natural self-healing process. If you open yourself to being curious without self-judgment, you're likely to get surprising feedback about what might have caused the interruption. What many people find when they work through this step is that some sort of situational, developmental, or environmental trauma holds the key to this diagnostic process. Many, though not all, illnesses may be the result of unhealed trauma, especially those mysterious illnesses that are either hard to diagnose, have no known treatment, or do not respond well to conventional medical treatment. Current life issues may be retriggering those early traumas and putting the body in a perpetual stress response. Those on a healing journey may also discover uncomfortable truths of how they have been out of integrity in their lives in ways that have hurt themselves and others. This can be a disruptive but illuminating and liberating step. Diagnosing these root causes prepares you to treat them in the next step, and when you dare to enter deep inquiry in this way, startling and life-changing revelations can enter your awareness as a gift of transformation.

Step Five: Write The Prescription for yourself. Tuning in to your Inner Pilot Light, allow yourself to be guided to the action steps that you intuit will help you heal the root causes you diagnosed in Step Four. Step Five may very well include conventional medical treatments, as well as other interventions. This inner doctor/therapist/healer will help you choose between conventional treatment options, as well as offer you action steps intended to restore your nervous system to a balanced state of homeostasis and healing. Your Inner Pilot Light might help you choose the right medical team and the optimal drug or surgery. You may be guided to start working with a trauma therapist or naturopath. You may *just know* it's time to heal or end your marriage, confront your boss, change careers, write the book you've dreamed of writing, set boundaries with a family member, do a green juice cleanse, or sign up for a yoga membership. Write it all down so you can see it all in one place. You may only know the first step, and that's fine. One intuitively guided action step may lead to the next, and if you trust the process, all you need to know is your next right step.

Step Six: Treat your fears and resistance. Before you attempt to take any action, you'll need to unblock any conscious or subconscious resistance. Otherwise, you'll be spinning your wheels, with one foot on the gas and one foot on the brake. If you find yourself resisting at least some part of this healing journey, you're not alone. Most people do. You might be afraid to follow through on what your Inner Pilot Light is guiding you to do. You might be subconsciously resistant to losing any hidden benefits you may be getting from being sick. You may also feel overwhelmed with a whole series of lifestyle changes and treatments that need to be implemented. You might be afraid of the financial consequences. You might worry about what other people will think or fear losing a valued relationship or the security it brings. You might even get uncomfortably flushed with intense emotions, even positive emotions, when you imagine what life might be like if you were one of those radical remissions at the end of all this. All of your resistance is welcome. Most of us have resistance to change, even positive change. Treating your resistance may take some guidance, requiring expert help, or your resistant parts might relax just because you give them permission to feel what they feel.

Now let's unpack each of the steps, and I'll share with you some of the practices you can use yourself or with clients.

Step One: Believe That Healing Is Possible.

What the placebo and nocebo data taught us is that if you're plagued by negative, self-sabotaging beliefs about your health, either consciously or subconsciously, any attempt to heal may be hampered by the limitations of your beliefs. At least a certain percentage of the time, what you believe manifests in the body. Most people believe certain illnesses are incurable, terminal, or chronic, but what if such beliefs are simply false?

For a long time, people believed that it was physiologically impossible for a human being to run a mile in less than four minutes. As long as everybody believed it to be true, nobody ever ran a sub-four-minute mile. Then something radical happened.

In 1954, Roger Bannister proved the sports physiologists wrong by running the mile in 3 minutes and 59 seconds for the first time in recorded history. Suddenly, the worldwide belief that running a sub-four-minute mile was physiologically impossible disappeared. Shortly thereafter, several other runners went on to run a mile in less than four minutes. In one famous race only 46 days later, Roger Bannister and John Landy both ran the mile in under four minutes, with Bannister winning the race.

Leading up to this time, athletes had been running faster and faster, but the four-minute mark seemed to erect a real physiological barrier nobody could overcome. It's as if the body simply couldn't cross over because the mind held this belief. But as soon as the belief was shattered by Bannister, the body was able to accomplish seemingly miraculous feats of athleticism.

Now, with the limiting belief that it was physiologically impossible shattered, virtually every athlete who competes in a world-class event has run the mile in under four minutes. Today's world-record time for the mile is 3:43:15, more than 15 seconds under 4 minutes.

What if believing that certain diseases cannot be cured is simply a limiting belief like the one that limited the athletes who longed to break the four-minute mile? What if you changed that self-sabotaging belief and allowed for the possibility that you, like the people whose medical miracles were reported in the Spontaneous Remission Project and the cancer patients Kelly Turner studied, might be free of what others might consider an incurable illness?

Just like the athletes who couldn't run the sub-four-minute mile—and then did—you may be held back by beliefs that are limiting what your body can do. As long as you believe your disease is incurable, this may be a self-fulfilling prophecy. But what if simply changing your mind could alter your brain, while simultaneously altering your body's physiology?

Remember the meditating monks who could visualize a fire in their bellies and increase their body temperatures? You, too, can change your physiology with the power of your consciousness. It helps to start with meditation. Quieting your mind makes it more receptive to changing beliefs. Try using the relaxation response or other meditation techniques described in Chapter 8 as preparation for other belief-changing practices.

Let me invite you to open your mind. Make room for the "impossible." You just never know what miracles might happen. To shift into a frequency of possibility, it helps to gift yourself with a full sensory experience of what your life might be like if your illness was gone. What would you be capable of doing that you can't do now? How would you celebrate your miracle? What dreams would you pursue? What delight might you relish? Give yourself a virtual experience by savoring what is possible.

Step One Exercise: Savor What's Possible

1. Close your eyes and let your imagination go wild with delight. Imagine that cure might be in the cards for you, even if others have told you to give up hope. What would that feel like? What would you do that you can't do now? What emotions would you feel if you were free of all suffering? How would your body feel? How would your heart feel? What prayer of gratitude would you say? How would you celebrate? Who would celebrate with you?

2. Let yourself have an inner experience "as if." Spend at least 15 minutes fully letting your inner world feel like you're cured. Make it as real as you possibly can to shift yourself internally from the dense emotions of sickness and disease to the more elevated feelings of celebration of a miracle.

3. Repeat this as often as you remember to do so, giving yourself the emotions and inner vision of what might be possible for you if cure is available to you.

Because many of our beliefs are like computer programs running in the background, hidden from our conscious awareness, it can be challenging to know how to ferret out beliefs that might be sabotaging optimal health. The following exercise is intended to help you bring into conscious awareness beliefs that might be unconscious. Before engaging in this exercise, try asking your intuition to help you heal by helping you identify negative core beliefs that might need to be shifted.

Step One Exercise: Examine Your Beliefs About Health

Write down the answers to these questions in your journal.

- What are my beliefs about health in general?
- What do I believe about my genetics and how my genes affect my health?
- What are my beliefs about my illness?
- Do I believe I need to be sick in order to get my needs met?
- What did my parents teach me about health, illness, or how healing happens?
- What are my beliefs about the body's ability to repair itself?
- What are my beliefs about my mind's effect on my body?
- Am I open to exploring that the root cause of my illness is not purely physical? If not, why not?
- What do I gain from my illness?
- Am I willing to give up what I gain from my illness in order to get well?
- Am I worthy of optimal health?

If you've been told your whole life that you're a sickly child or that cancer runs in your family, these beliefs will anchor in your system and predispose you to actually being sickly or getting cancer. To live an optimally healthy life, such beliefs need to be shifted. Otherwise, you're likely to wind up like the runners who were unable to run a four minute mile until their limiting beliefs were shattered.

But what actually works to shift beliefs? You've probably noticed that positive affirmations have limited efficacy. It would be great if you could just chant "I am enough" and be free of all those beliefs about worthlessness, unlovability, and inadequacy, in addition to all your limiting beliefs about health. But to truly transform negative beliefs into positive ones, you have to treat the traumas that caused the beliefs in the first place. Because most of us were traumatized in ways that made us feel insignificant, unworthy, and not enough, no amount of repeating an affirmation will treat the core wounds that made you believe you weren't enough to begin with. Trying to change your beliefs at the level of the conscious mind has little efficacy because you are only operating from your conscious mind 5 percent of the time. This is why repeating affirmations usually have little effect, because the minute you revert to the limiting beliefs running on autopilot in the subconscious mind, your affirmations get negated.

So what does work? The traditional therapeutic approach to changing your beliefs is the "cognitive" part of Cognitive Behavioral Therapy (CBT). In essence, you can argue with or dispute your thoughts, catching yourself when you have a belief or thought, then actively stopping the belief or thought and replacing it with a healthier one. This cognitive gymnastics takes vigilance and mindfulness, since most negative thoughts and beliefs run on autopilot and must be interrupted in order for this process to be helpful

Byron Katie's "The Work" is similar to CBT. This process of inquiry invites you to ask four questions based on a painful thought or belief—Is it true? Can you absolutely know that it's true? How do you react, what happens, when you believe that thought? Who would you be without that thought? Then you're invited to replace that thought or belief with the "turnaround," a healthier, restorative thought or belief.

While some people benefit from cognitive approaches like this, and CBT has been shown to improve functioning in patients with depression and anxiety, many studies show that improvements in mood do not necessarily reduce the painful automatic thoughts that stem from negative core beliefs. Like affirmations, CBT has been shown to have limited efficacy when it comes to changing the automatic negative thinking that negative core beliefs activate.[1]

The good news is that the field of psychotherapy is growing to include energetic clearing methods that seem to work better. Emotional Freedom Techniques (EFT, or Tapping) is the energy psychology method with the largest database of research behind it, validating its efficacy as treatment for a variety of conditions that are often accompanied by negative core beliefs, including PTSD.[2,3] Many patients and practitioners are using this easy-to-learn self-help tool for clearing limiting beliefs and uploading healthier belief programs into the subconscious mind.

Although there is not yet scientific evidence to support its efficacy, my favorite tool for clearing trauma and shifting the negative core beliefs that accompany it is Advanced Integrative Therapy (AIT), an energy psychotherapy created by Asha Clinton, Ph.D., my personal therapist. The AIT model first identifies and clears whatever trauma caused the negative core belief, then energetically and somatically removes the belief, replacing it with a restorative, healing belief that is its realistic, positive opposite. The reason AIT Core Belief work is so powerful is that this psychotherapeutic model treats the traumas that cause the problematic core beliefs before treating the core beliefs themselves. While many other psychotherapies, such as CBT, focus on symptom relief, AIT recognizes that treating a symptom, such as a problematic core belief, doesn't remove it permanently, whereas treating the trauma that caused the dysfunctional core belief and then treating the relationship between the trauma and the belief creates lasting healing of both. As with any psychotherapy, self-help practices are not as effective as working directly with an AIT therapist. But if you're burdened with negative core beliefs, the following practice may grant you some relief.

Step One Exercise: Clear Negative Core Beliefs with Advanced Integrative Therapy (AIT)

To review a video of this AIT negative core belief clearing technique, download the Self-Healing Kit at MindOverMedicine Book.com.

1. Identify the negative core beliefs that you discovered in the "Examine Your Beliefs about Health" exercise. Examples of health-related negative core beliefs include:

   - *I need to get sick in order to get love and attention.*
   - *I have to be sick in order to not deplete myself caretaking others.*
   - *My body betrayed me.*

2. Identify the realistic positive opposite. For example:

   - *I can have love and attention without staying sick.*
   - *I can choose not to caretake others and be well.*
   - *My body was betrayed.*

3. Identify how true the negative core belief is. On a scale of zero to ten, where zero means you don't believe the negative belief at all and ten means it is 100 percent true for you, how strongly do you believe this negative belief now? Pick the number that feels intuitively true to you.

4. Remove the negative belief by moving your hand down the energy centers, one by one. You can observe where these energy centers are on the video. Repeat the negative core belief as you touch each energy center.

5. Close your eyes and check inside. On a scale of zero to ten, how true does the statement still feel?

6. If your number is anything above zero, repeat the sequence and keep going until you experience the negative core belief at a zero. If you're having trouble getting to zero, there may be an underlying trauma that needs to be treated before you're ready to let go of that core belief. An AIT therapist can help you get to

the root of what might be interfering with your ability to clear it.

7. Once the negative core belief is at a zero, you are ready to install the new realistic positive belief. Feel into how true the new belief feels. On a scale of zero to ten, where zero means that you don't believe the new positive core belief at all, and where ten means that you totally believe it, pick a number.

8. Install the new belief at each energy center. While clearing beliefs requires moving down the energy centers, you'll move upward as you install new beliefs, starting at the root (perineum) and moving up to the crown (top of your head). Repeat the positive core belief at each center, moving at your own pace from root to crown.

9. When you reach the crown, on a scale of zero to ten, check into how true the new statement feels. If it's less than ten, do another round.

10. When you reach ten, having installed the new belief maximally, say "Hallelujah!" or whatever other form of celebration feels resonant with you. Feel the gratitude for the important work you've just done.

Note: If you were doing this with an AIT therapist, muscle testing would be used to verify that your intuition is accurately interpreting how true the belief is, as well as when it's cleared/installed successfully. While teaching the AIT method of muscle testing is beyond the scope of this book, if you know how to muscle test, you can test yourself or have a friend or practitioner double-check your intuition.

Step Two: Connect and Surrender to Your Inner Pilot Light, Letting Your Inner Knowing Guide Your Healing Journey.

Step Two is about cultivating internal support. Every single one of us has the perfect healer within. Step Two invites you to connect with this intuitive aspect of your being, trust it, and surrender to it. You wouldn't be here if there wasn't something you yearn to heal. Longing for change, whether the change you seek is relief from physical pain, mental suffering, restoration of full function, a longer life, clearing trauma, or spiritual awakening, is the fuel that activates most healing journeys. This longing is a gift, since it serves as the catalyst to bring you closer to the mysterious forces that can help guide you and restore you to wholeness.

Yet before you even begin this journey, let's begin with the humble acknowledgment that you are not in control of this journey. This is a curious paradox. You are an empowered patient, taking your power back and doing what you can to make your body ripe for miracles, *and* you are not in control of how this journey will go or what its outcome will be. The simple act of offering your journey to your Inner Pilot Light—or to God, the Divine, or the Universe—sets the stage for allowing yourself to enter a flow state that can carry you on this journey, rather than requiring you to swim upstream. This is not a passive act or a way of giving up. This practice of surrendering to a spiritual Source invokes a mysterious process that you'll have to experience yourself, one that you don't have to be religious or buy into any belief to experience. Surrendering to a force beyond your small self is a numinous, ineffable experience of humbly asking to be guided to whatever will support you best on your journey.

In my Christian upbringing, I was taught to pray for what you want. Every Sunday, the pastor dutifully read off the list of prayer requests and we all prayed for God to help these suffering people get what they wanted. But my spiritual mentor taught me to pray a bit differently. When she was about to have surgery, she asked her surgeon if he would pray with her. He said, "Of course. Shall we pray for a good outcome?"

She said, "No, let us pray for that which is most right."

Her surgeon told her afterward that he had never felt such a powerful presence in the operating room. "The minute we said that prayer, all of my anxiety and all the pressure I felt about operating on someone I respect so much vanished. It's like something larger than me was using my hands and my mind to orchestrate the most effortless, perfect surgery I've ever performed. I just knew that, even if you had died on the table, I was being used to serve whatever was most right."

How would it feel to surrender to this kind of prayer? *Let us pray for that which is most right.* This practice invites us into the humble awareness that what is most right is a mystery. It's a way to offer your body and your healing to whatever force of love you trust. Imagine that the force of love that created you is an intimate partner in your healing journey, and you won't want to do anything or make any decision without consulting this Beloved first, just as you would a spouse or close friend.

Some people resist the notion of spiritual surrender because of spiritual traumas they've experienced from spiritually disconnected atheist parents or judging, even abusive people who were part of their religious upbringing. Even in 12-step programs for people who are in recovery from addictions or codependent relationships with addicts, some of the biggest resistance comes from the steps that ask participants to turn their lives over to "God as we understood Him;" some people are allergic to the word *God* or triggered by the pronoun *Him* or generally attached to the belief that spirituality is the opiate of the masses. From my point of view, the language and the gender pronouns are irrelevant to this process, and the kind of mystical spirituality I'm referring to is free of any religious dogma. I have found that while some people have a deep and abiding faith in a traditional religious deity—and this is fine—many people are more willing to surrender to the divine spark inside each of us, because it's not hampered by any outdated religious hang-ups or power trips. Your connection to the spark of divinity within you is your birthright, but maybe people have spent most of their lives disconnected from it. Restoring this connection is essential to the healing process.

What Is Your Inner Pilot Light?

Here's how I describe it in my book *The Daily Flame: 365 Love Letters from Your Inner Pilot Light.*

Every life begins when a small spark of the Eternal Flame of cosmic consciousness splits off like a glowing ember of a universal bonfire. This unique spark ignites as the Organizing Intelligence that creates your organs, divides your cells, and develops you perfectly into a precious being decorated with thoughts, preferences, gifts, talents, emotions, and eccentricities. Your Inner Pilot Light begins in every baby as the untainted, radiant, buoyant light of God/Goddess but often gets filmed over by trauma, conditioning, and the illusion of separation from the Eternal Flame from which this unique spark arises. Although your Inner Pilot Light may grow dim as life's inevitable challenges threaten to snuff out the full brilliance of this luminous fire, rest assured that your Inner Pilot Light never burns out. Even when you die, the spark returns to the Eternal Flame, adding the brilliance of this unique fractal of light to that which creates all life.

In mystical moments, you may be graced with a glimpse through the film that veils your Inner Pilot Light, experiencing moments of enlivening ecstasy, bliss, and unity as your unique flame merges with the bonfire of all life. Yet, this veil usually creeps back in like fog pouncing into a valley between coastal mountains off a cool ocean, cooling the luminous flames and quieting the burn back to an ember. When the fog retreats back to sea and your Inner Pilot Light flares up, you may have moments of clear vision, deep knowing, and a true remembering of the Oneness that links us all. Then the fog rolls back in, and you may forget once again that your singular flame is also part of the One bonfire.

Over time, the fog may roll in less, and the fire within you may gain fuel from the practices that connect you to the Eternal Flame, stoking your inner fire with your devotion, your discipline, your prayers, your humility, and your longing to reconnect with that which once burst you into life. As you peel away all that is not love to allow more oxygen to fan the flames of consciousness in your original spark, as the inevitable trauma of human life heals, and as the center of your love is unveiled, this flame within you grows to fill your cells. This original spark fills your whole body until it bleeds through your skin as an invisible field of love that touches the spaces around you, lending this warmth to all who come near.

It's not easy to get the mind to loosen its stronghold on attempts to control your life, especially if you're sick and scared. But just as addicts might need to hit rock bottom before they're willing to admit that they have lost control, sometimes we need to hit rock bottom through the physical body in order to cede control to a larger aspect of our being. In *An Untethered Soul,* Michael Singer writes about the nature of our relationship to the human mind. "You said to your mind, 'I want everyone to like me. I don't want anyone to speak badly of me. I want everything I say and do to be pleasing and acceptable to everyone. I don't want anyone to hurt me. I don't want anything to happen that I don't like. And I want everything to happen that I do like.' Then you said, 'Now mind, go figure out how to make every one of these things a reality, even if you have to think about it day and night.' And of course your mind says, 'I'm on the job. I will work on it constantly.'"

This is why the practice of spiritual surrender is a constant practice. It's not something you do once and then forget about it. It's a journey, an ever-deepening trust in something larger than the small, local mind. The way I think about it, surrendering to this "something larger" is a way of getting beyond the protector parts of the mind, the parts that are always busy thinking about how to get you what you want and avoid what you don't want. You're really surrendering the local mind to what some would call "non-local mind" or the "One Mind." By relaxing into this trust, you are casting the burden of figuring out life to this organizing intelligence, which has a wider perspective and a powerful ability to orchestrate what is needed to bring about that which is most right.

This practice also has a powerful side effect. What I've found from years of facilitating this practice with patients and health-care providers, as well as practicing it myself, is that painful, angst-ridden emotions associated with grasping for something you don't yet have tend to release, sometimes through tears and sometimes through primal noises or physical movements. On an emotional level, the end result of this practice is a deep, abiding, gratitude-inducing peace, the kind of relief that relaxes the nervous system and activates your self-healing mechanisms right away. Your healing has begun, before you've actually *done* anything.

206

Unlike many "law of attraction" or manifestation practices that are aimed at leveraging your spiritual power to get you what you want, this is not about getting what you want, although the manifestation of your desire is a common, unexpected, and seemingly miraculous outcome. It's about letting go of what you want and dissolving into the desire to live in alignment with that which is most right, whatever that might be. A common outcome, paradoxically, is that you get what you want after all, or you get the *feeling* of what you thought you wanted, but it shows up in a way you might never have expected. It can feel quite magical, the way things tend to work out in a way your mind would never have imagined.

People talk about spiritual surrender as this exalted practice of letting go of the illusion of control, but few people talk about the *"how"* of surrender. Meeting Tosha Silver changed my entire relationship to spiritual surrender, and I want to share with you one of the most profound surrendering practices she taught me. It's called the God Box Meditation, and I facilitate this exercise in every live event I teach. One of my physician clients had a profound experience during the God Box Meditation. She had tried every form of infertility treatment in her attempt to get pregnant, depleting her emotional, physical, and financial resources. But her yearning to become a mother was so strong, she couldn't give up, and continued obsessing over getting pregnant. Surrendering this primal desire to becoming a mother during the God Box Meditation evoked an intense emotional catharsis that opened her to a new lightness of being. She suddenly felt free, like she no longer had to become a mother through her own womb in order to live a deep, fulfilling life. She realized she could adopt a child, or maybe she wasn't even meant to adopt. For the first time in her life, she trusted "that which is most right" and was able to let go of her painful obsession with getting what she wanted. Because her mind relaxed, she was able to follow the flow of what came next. She felt guided to do just one more cycle with her infertility doctor, and shazaam! She got pregnant within a month of the God Box ceremony. About this experience, she said, "When I let go of my attachment to what I wanted so desperately and trusted in allowing that which is right and highest to occur, everything flowed. The practice of surrender continued throughout my pregnancy. Even though my physical body was carrying the child, I felt like a vessel and that a force unseen to me was taking care of both of us."

Unexpected outcomes like these are common side effects of this practice, though there are no guarantees. Letting go of the need for any sort of guaranteed outcome is foundational to the practice. Tosha Silver says, "The very act of grasping for the feather creates the wind current that pushes it away." When you let go of attachment to outcomes, that which is meant for you can float to you effortlessly and that which is not meant for you will float on by, leaving you in peace, even if you don't get what you want.

As you begin this healing journey, I invite you to experience this practice for yourself.

Step Two Exercise: Offer Your Healing to "The God Box"

1. Prepare for this practice by finding any kind of box you wish to represent your God Box. It could be as simple as a shoebox, or you may feel drawn to something more ornate that you'll keep on an altar. Your God Box might also exist only in your mind's eye, and this is fine, but it can anchor the practice to tie it to a physical release.

2. Begin by closing your eyes and putting your attention on the center of your heart, breathing in and out through your heart as you do, focusing on a feeling of gratitude that your Inner Pilot Light is here to be with you to help support this practice. Breathe this gratitude in and out through your heart, feeling as if what you deeply desire has already come true. Allow yourself to imagine that you are fully and completely healed. How would that feel? Call in those emotions now.

3. Visualize a temple in the center of your heart. Observe it, feel it, smell it, taste it. See a God Box, something you will surrender your desire into, sitting on an altar in the temple inside your heart. In this place

of serenity, allow yourself to call in a presence you will surrender with. It may be a deity, an ancestor, an animal spirit, an angel, a redwood tree, or your Inner Pilot Light, as long as it represents the unknowable force of love that will be with you through this practice. Let yourself feel comforted by this grounded, unconditionally loving presence.

4. Allow yourself to feel the vulnerability of three things that tend to keep the mind busy—unmet longings, unsolved problems, and undecided decisions. Make a list with three columns—unmet longings, unsolved problems, and undecided decisions. Open your eyes just long enough to write down these items, but do not lose the sensation of being inside the temple in your heart, in the comfort of this being of love, who is here to help you surrender. Your unmet longings might include a cure for your illness, a life partner if you're single, the money to buy your freedom from a job you hate, or getting pregnant if you've been infertile. Your unsolved problems might include a troubled marriage, a conflict at work, or how to deal with an addict child. Your undecided decisions might include treatment decisions, the decision to change careers, or the decision to enter couple's therapy.

5. After completing your lists, close your eyes again and enter the temple inside your heart. Let yourself cast this burden of all the heaviness of what's on your lists into the great arms of love offered by the being that is here to take these burdens from you. Let yourself feel whatever arises—grief, sadness, disappointment, despair, relief, gratitude, lightness of being. It's all welcome. Notice how you feel when this being of love takes these burdens, puts your list in the God Box for you, and says to you, "Sweetheart, I've got this. You don't need to worry about it anymore. Let me handle it my way."

6. Now let yourself feel the feelings you would feel if everything you just put in the God Box was handled. How would you feel if all your longings came true— or if you simply stopped longing for whatever wasn't "most right" for you on your journey to wholeness? What if your problems were suddenly, mysteriously solved? What if you knew with perfect clarity which decision to make? How would you feel then? As chiropractor Sue Morter writes in *The Energy Codes*, "*Wanting* has a different frequency than *having* does, so if we're in the vibration of wanting something, we're not going to have it." Let yourself have it with all your heart, soul, and body.

7. If you have a physical God Box, you can physically surrender your lists to the God Box as a somatic gesture of letting go. Tear up your list. Make it into a paper airplane and fly it in. Dance it to the God Box. You may even want to take the God Box to a ceremonial fire and burn the contents as an act of release.

8. You can do this practice without a physical God Box too. Your portable God Box lives forever now in the temple in your heart and you can surrender every time you find yourself perseverating on unmet longings, unsolved problems, and undecided decisions. The key to this practice is to remember to do it—over and over and over until it becomes second nature.

For an audio version of this God Box Meditation as well as many other tools for tuning in, register for the Connect to Your Inner Pilot Light program at InnerPilotLight.com.

Why does this practice work? For one thing, it shifts you from fear of uncertainty into curiosity, even excitement about the unknowable future that lies before you. When you don't know what the future holds, *anything* can happen, even a miracle. It also brings you into the present moment, which is the only place you can receive spiritual guidance intended to support the rest of your journey. If you're in your head, you're not in your body, in your direct experience, in the present, in a relaxed nervous system, or in your intuition. Surrendering opens you to the rest of the journey.

Step Three: Surround Yourself with Healing Support

Step Three is about cultivating external support. As previously discussed, although your body has the ability to repair itself when things break down, you won't want to navigate your healing journey solo. Not only will you need a well-trained facilitator to guide you through your psycho-spiritual healing process. You'll also want to optimize whatever potential treatments physicians and modern medicine have to offer as an adjunct to healing the disease-creating thoughts, beliefs, and feelings that emotional, mental, and spiritual trauma can induce. Whole Health requires a truly holistic approach. This is not about turning away from the miracles of modern science, nor is it about relying solely on conventional medicine to give you a hall pass from healing any underlying psychological, spiritual, or environmental trauma that may be causing or exacerbating your health condition. Whole Health is a marriage of both, leading to an intuitively guided treatment plan that only you can prescribe, which may include many different healing modalities. Those who you select to join you at the Healing Round Table are the practitioners and soul allies who will help support you through this journey.

How will you create the Healing Round Table, where you are responsible for inviting collaborative practitioners to join the table, and nobody has hierarchy over anyone else? Can you dare to take a stand for team members who can help you optimize your health outcome? And if your own past trauma is making it hard for you to do this, can you find someone who can help support you while you treat your own reluctance to take a stand for your healing? Here are a few invitations for inquiry which might help you choose.

Step Three Exercise: Examine Your Healing Support

Write the answers to these questions in your journal.

- How seen and heard do I feel by my health-care providers?

- What is my biggest fear about challenging a health-care provider or choosing someone else?

- Am I asking for what I need from my health-care providers? If not, why not?

- Are there any ways I'm sabotaging my own health care?

- How do I support my own health?

- How do I feel when I leave my health-care provider?

- What would make me feel better supported and more empowered in my relationships with my health-care providers?

- Am I fully disclosing what's true to my health-care provider? If not, why not?

- Am I worthy of sharing power with my health-care providers?

- What issues from my past might keep me from feeling able to partner with my health-care providers as an empowered patient?

- Am I asking my friends and family for help when I need it? If not, why not?

- What beliefs or tendencies, such as rugged individualism, lacking assertiveness, or giving my power away, may be interfering with my ability to build a team of healing support? What needs to be healed so I can transform my stuckness?

- Am I worth paying cash if I need help outside the traditional health-care system? What are my beliefs about money and health?

When embarking on a healing journey, it takes a village. How do you find the right team of people to sit at your Healing Round Table? Here are some guidelines.

- Interview your team. Let them know when you make the appointment that you would like to schedule a consultation to make sure the fit is right. If the doctor, therapist, or CAM provider won't submit to being interviewed, find someone who will. The right health-care providers will not be insulted by your request. But be prepared to pay out of pocket for such an interview. Your insurance may not cover it.

- Find health-care providers who believe in you. The scientific data suggests that if your health-care provider believes you have the potential to get well, you're more likely to thrive. Feel free to ask your provider flat out, "Do you believe I can get better?" Pay close attention to the answer. If your doctor reads you negative statistics, insists that the outlook is not good, labels you as "incurable," and generally considers you a hopeless case, you might think about finding someone else. Keep in mind that as physicians, we are trained to be "realists" (a.k.a. "pessimists"), so don't write off physicians who are skeptical right away. Many people who have read this book have offered the practitioners they selected as part of their Healing Round Table a copy of *Mind Over Medicine* and asked them if they'd be willing to read it and partner on a healing journey. While some won't have the time or interest in doing so, many patients have reported that their practitioners, including their doctors, were thrilled to enter into a healing partnership like this after receiving a copy of *Mind Over Medicine* from an inquiring patient. I've also been told that some practitioners are giving out this book to patients, inviting them to participate on their end in order to achieve better collaborative health outcomes. While not every provider will be on board for this approach to a healing journey, those who are will be grateful to work in partnership. Your participation takes a lot of pressure off them!

- Seek health-care providers who truly care. It's time to bring the "care" back to health care. You are more than a room number or a body part. If your provider can't treat you like the whole, fabulous human being you are, keep looking and find someone who can. There are loads of talented, nurturing practitioners with remarkable skills, excellent bedside manners, and big, wide-open hearts just waiting for a wonderful patient like you.

- Put your body in the hands of providers willing to collaborate. If your homeopath hates doctors, and your doctor thinks your Reiki master is a quack, it's going to be hard to get everyone on the same page. If you're assembling a team that includes healers outside the scope of conventional medicine, make sure your providers are willing and eager to communicate respectfully with each other so you don't wind up getting conflicting advice that not only confuses you, but can be downright dangerous.

- Listen to the wisdom of your body. What does your gut say when you're with your health-care provider? Do you feel safe in her hands? Do you trust him? Do you think you'll get sound medical advice or do you get a weird vibe? Check in with how your body reacts. If you feel tight, clenched, nervous, cold, shivery, or closed off, your body may be telling you something. Look for feelings of openness, warmth, relaxation, and calmness in your body.

- Make sure your health-care provider respects your intuition. If you question a treatment and express your opinion in a respectful manner and your intuition isn't respected, you might think twice about whether this is the best provider for you. As health-care providers, our job is to present you with your options, educate you about the risks and benefits, and make treatment recommendations, but ultimately, the choice is 100 percent yours. If your practitioner gets her panties in a wad because you don't choose to follow her recommendations, it's her problem, not yours. The right practitioner will welcome your feedback, understand that you know your body better than anybody else, and respect your wishes.

- Be willing to sign a waiver. In today's litigious society, your practitioners or their malpractice-insurance carriers may require that you sign a waiver if you opt to decline the treatment they recommend but still wish to be a patient under their care. Don't take it personally. They're just covering their butts, and it doesn't mean that they don't support your autonomy.

- Know that you deserve the best care possible. Don't go telling yourself stories about how you're not good enough/smart enough/ young enough/rich enough/[fill in the blank] enough to get this kind of stellar medical care. You may have to pay out of pocket to get it, since some forward-thinking doctors have opted out of the insurance system in order to offer premium health care and more time with patients. But what is more important than your health? If you can afford to give up other luxuries and pay out of pocket for top-notch health care, please do.

- Seek out a Whole Health Medicine Institute graduate. Our graduates have all been trained to show up this way in a healing partnership. They've also been trained to facilitate the Six Steps to Healing Yourself. You can find Whole Health Medicine Institute graduates under the "find professional" tab at WholeHealthMedicineInstitute.com.

Your Community of Healing

In the last decade since I began researching my first version of *Mind Over Medicine* and followed up with *Sacred Medicine*, society has changed dramatically. With the increased usage of technology, especially handheld devices, and social media, people are spending more time by ourselves, "connecting" virtually, and less time gathering together in real, live community. We are experiencing an epidemic of loneliness, fear of missing out, and dissatisfaction and uneasiness with our lives like never before. This overarching dis-ease with life has increased and intensified the amount of chronic disease, trauma, and injury we are burdened with. For many, it is harder than ever to achieve the relaxed states our nervous systems so critically need to achieve Whole Health and optimal healing.

In addition to the growing trend in disconnection, health-care costs have risen, disposable income has decreased, and people are struggling and are at a loss for how to find relief. At the same time, the wellness industry is booming, awareness about trauma healing and its relationship to Whole Health is increasing, and the number of people who identify as "spiritual but not religious" is on the rise. Yet as much as it might appear to be a reassuring sign that wellness, cutting-edge psychotherapies, spirituality, and many forms of natural healing are gaining in popularity, it's also true that these industries (and make no mistake, they're multibillion-dollar industries) have been hijacked by consumerism and commoditized as luxury goods. Few of the wellness modalities described in this book are covered by insurance or public aid, leaving these opportunities for healing available only to the elite, while millions of others either can't afford the kind of care they need or don't even know it exists. On the other hand, many of those who do have excess income often don't have the right doctors, therapists, healers, spiritual counselors, educational tools, or Whole Health–inducing practices to overcome their personal health challenges, leaving even the privileged minority with chronic and sometimes life-threatening health or disability issues.

In response to this cultural and healing crisis, I became inspired to do something about it and founded Heal At Last, a novel solution that addresses the epidemic of loneliness, the need for affordable, scalable, and diversity-inclusive communities of healing, and a way to reach otherwise financially disadvantaged, marginalized, and motivated individuals so they can employ psycho-spiritual healing methods together, in community. Heal At Last is the social justice, philanthropic, and public health arm of the body of healing work represented in *Mind Over Medicine*, which brings together healing modalities from a variety of traditions, synthesizing them into a program that serves those in recovery from illness, injury, or trauma in a similar way to how 12-step programs serve those in recovery from addictions. At Heal At Last, we are creating community-driven transformational healing circles both online and in person that are led by professionally trained leaders.

Imagine being in a group, something like an Alcoholics Anonymous meeting, in a living room, hospital, church, or community center near you, filled with open-minded, spiritually curious, judgment-free, diversity-inclusive, wellness-motivated friends and allies. But instead of sinking into your victim stories, the way support groups can sometimes devolve, this healing circle has an uplifting vibe, bubbling with possibilities and soul-infused effervescence. Instead of standing up and speaking about your addiction, you share with others how your illness, injury, or trauma is holding you back from living a thriving life. In addition, you get to engage in group healing practices to transform whatever you are struggling with into meaning, depth, intimacy, and healing, alchemizing your adversity into an opportunity for growth and awakening. You also commit to yourself and your group to embark on the journey to Whole Health together, since consistency and commitment to a group has proven to be the cornerstone of positive change, as other recovery programs have shown. As the scientific data demonstrates, it's also one of the keys to healing loneliness, a major risk factor for disease and impediment to healing.

Your healing circle not only serves as a kind and compassionate witness to your journey, which is very soul nourishing in itself; it also provides support and feedback on how to move through your health challenge to achieve a state of ongoing recovery, to decrease your likelihood of replacing one physical or mental health crisis with the next one. The goal is to help your health span equal your lifespan. The foundation of the meetings is based not only on the Six Steps to Healing Yourself, but also on other healing modalities not usually included in conventional medical treatment.

Heal At Last has a goal to be affordable, accessible, and safe for all people, regardless of income, race, religion, sexual orientation, or political affiliation. If you are in need of healing, are a healer interested in volunteering your gifts to those in need, or are a philanthropist and would like to participate in funding our programs, visit HealAtLast.org to learn more. This is a grassroots effort, and it will take a village to realize our vision. We welcome you to join our movement.

If Heal At Last doesn't feel right for you, start your own healing circle! Don't be afraid to reach out to your friends and let them know you need love, support, nurture, play time, help with whatever tasks you might be unable to do, time with others out in nature, music, dancing, and healing touch. So often, people who are sick have a hard time asking for and receiving care. Think of your illness as a way to help you learn how to get your needs met, but once you learn the lesson your illness can help you learn, get your needs met in ways that don't require you to be sick in order to get love, nurture, and support. Don't grow dependent on getting or being sick in order to learn that you deserve a tribe of loving people who, like the people of Roseto, Pennsylvania, can help you navigate the vicissitudes of life. If reaching out to others to ask for support feels daunting, find a meet up of like-minded people who share a common interest—art, meditation, spiritual beliefs, hiking, or even guinea pigs! (I'm not kidding. One woman I knew joined a guinea pig club as part of her healing journey.) You can find or start just about any gathering of like-minded people on MeetUp.com.

Step Four: Diagnose the Root Causes of Your Illness

If you have a health condition, your doctor may have already given you a diagnosis—angina, Crohn's disease, diabetes, breast cancer, whatever. As I've said before, if you're experiencing symptoms and haven't yet seen a doctor, please get to it—pronto. We've come a long way in the past century, and modern medicine has much to offer, so it's crucial to find out if your doctor can offer curative treatment options. (Remember: you can always investigate your options and then choose to say no to those treatment options. It's your body, your life, your choice.)

But what if you've seen five doctors, you have a medical chart three inches thick, and in spite of everyone's best efforts, nobody has been able to figure out what's wrong with you? What if you've got a diagnosis, but no curative treatment is known for your particular condition? If you're one of those frustrated patients whom doctors haven't been able to give a diagnosis or treat adequately, don't despair. Sometimes your diagnosis is right around the corner, and it's just a matter of seeing the right physician. But other times, a conventional medical diagnosis simply doesn't exist, or a curative treatment has not yet been discovered. The good news is that having symptoms with no diagnosis or having a diagnosis conventional medicine doesn't know how to cure may make you a great candidate for having a remarkable outcome using the Six Steps to Healing Yourself.

It's not that your symptoms are "all in your head," because clearly, they're in your body. But when you're experiencing symptoms your doctor can't diagnose or adequately treat, it's often because the symptoms are the result of repetitive triggering of the stress response without adequate relaxation-response counterbalancing. Conventional medicine simply doesn't yet have a catchall diagnosis for that physiological cascade of symptom-inducing effects.

Whether you have a traditional diagnosis, you're experiencing symptoms nobody can diagnose, or you're healthy but interested in preventive health, chances are good that you're not optimizing your body's capacity for self-repair and improving your chance of cure. That's where the next step in this process comes in. Almost every illness is either caused by or exacerbated by triggering of the stress response, which happens in the body but starts in the mind. While you can mitigate some of the stress response without understanding what's triggering it, you're better off digging deep and diagnosing the root cause of *what is triggering those stress responses in the first place.* If you're engaging in stress-relieving activities, such as meditation, creative expression, sex, yoga, or exercise, but you're not alleviating the source of the stress, you're not optimizing your body's chance for cure. If, however, you can heal the problem from the root and stop the stress response at its origin, you're much more likely to wind up cured.

When you diagnose the root causes of what is triggering your stress responses, you gain insight into how your body may be suffering as the result of your mind and how you can not only prevent future stress responses but initiate natural relaxation responses that have been proven to prevent and cure disease. Remember, prevention is always better than treatment, especially given that some manifestations of chronic stress in the body may be hard (though not impossible) for the body to undo after the fact.

While it may be too late to prevent an illness that already affects you, it's never too late to reduce stress responses and activate relaxation responses. While results vary and some conditions are more susceptible than others to reductions in stress responses and increases in relaxation, when you mobilize the body's natural mechanisms of self-repair, anything is possible and radical remission just might happen, even when you've been told your condition is chronic or incurable.

Before I move on to a series of exercises aimed at helping you identify what might be triggering your stress responses, let me say a few words about blame, shame, and guilt, which often come up when you initiate a conversation about root causes of illness or suggest that people might have the power to heal themselves. When I tell you that you might have the power to heal yourself, and when you realize that something within your control may be causing or exacerbating a health condition, you may be inclined to either kick yourself or kick me. Since I'd prefer to avoid both outcomes, let me officially declare this a blame/shame/guilt-free zone.

Being sick doesn't mean you've necessarily done anything wrong. It doesn't always mean you're the victim of sheer bad luck. Somewhere in the middle lies the truth. Clearly, there are dozens of factors that play into why one person gets sick and another doesn't or why one patient experiences radical remission and another stays sick. Contributing factors include the beliefs of the conscious and subconscious mind; the right health-care providers; diet and exercise; exposures to drugs, alcohol, tobacco, and environmental toxins; self-care habits; feeling loved and worthy; being happy; practices that initiate the relaxation response, and spiritual factors I won't get into here.

Clearly you have a lot of control over how healthy you are. If you're a three-pack-a-day smoker who winds up with lung cancer, you've been eating at McDonald's every day and get a heart attack, you've been boozing it up for three decades and wind up with cirrhosis of the liver, or you've stayed in an abusive marriage for so long that you get an autoimmune disease, it's clear that your lifestyle choices are probably affecting the health of your body.

But things also happen to your body that are completely out of your control. You're born with an extra chromosome. Your car is hit by a drunk driver. You unwittingly move in next to a toxic-waste dump. You're the victim of a drive-by shooting. The rebounder trampoline you're bouncing on snaps closed while you're bouncing on it and breaks your wrist.

Shit happens.

Whether your illness came about because you smoked too much, drank too much, overate, exposed yourself to toxic relationships, stayed in a soul-sucking job, left untreated trauma simmering in your cells, or were just plain unlucky, there's no point berating yourself for past events you can't change. Doing so will only trigger stress responses and make things worse.

But there is a place for personal responsibility. As Dr. Christiane Northrup once said to me when we were discussing this issue, "We are responsible *to* our disease, not *for* our disease."

I agree with her. Illness offers us a precious opportunity to investigate our lives without judgment, diagnose the root cause of what might be contributing to an illness, realign ourselves psychologically and spiritually, and do what we can to make our bodies ripe for miracles. When viewed with compassion and without judgment, illness can be a potent opportunity for personal growth and spiritual awakening.

Keep in mind as you navigate this process that your Inner Pilot Light, the wise healer that lies within you, is your body's best friend and always knows exactly what your body needs. But many have unwittingly distanced themselves from the wisdom of their Inner Pilot Lights. Often, this is because we no longer reside in our own bodies. Instead of living embodied lives, heeding the wisdom of our intuition, and feeling all five senses in our own skin, we dissociate. Doctors know this better than anyone. As a physician-in-training, I was expected to work almost constantly, so I wasn't free to sleep when I was tired, eat when I was hungry, pee when my bladder was full, quit operating when my shoulders got sore, or stay home and rest when I was sick. I had to soldier on, no matter what my body was telling me.

I was also too busy to listen to the quiet whispers of my intuitive knowing. Usually, I had to get whacked upside the head with the proverbial two-by-four. My body had to yell before I would notice that I had gotten off track in my life. As a defense against recurrent pain and discomfort, I learned to be a walking cerebrum, living in the vicinity of my body, but not fully in it. While doctors may be extreme examples of how we learn to stay in our minds and get out of our bodies so we don't experience physical or emotional pain, most of us experience some level of mind-body dissociation as an adaptation that later comes around to bite us. When we dissociate from the body, we don't hear the whispers the body delivers as warning signs intended to gently coax us into shape. We also get cut off from the "yes" and "no" feelings inside our bodies when we're making decisions that are in or out of alignment for our highest good, including health decisions.

But you can change all that. If you're having trouble tapping into the healing wisdom of your Inner Pilot Light, try using your body as a brilliant entry point into your intuition about what will help your body heal. When you learn to listen to the wisdom your body is sharing with you, you will find all the answers you need in order to navigate your self-healing journey. You'll also learn how to prevent future illness by noticing the whispers from your body before they become rebel yells. (For 8 tips on how to be in your body, see Appendix A.)

Remember, before you go through these diagnostic exercises, make sure you have the right support. We're about to get down and dirty, and I want to make sure you feel safe, loved, and nurtured, not just by someone else, but especially by yourself. With that in mind, let me walk you through a few exercises I use with patients to help them diagnose the root causes contributing to an illness.

Diagnostic Exercise #1: Let Your Body Be Your Guide

1. Get quiet. Spend a few moments sitting down, closing your eyes.

2. Breathe deeply. Notice your chest as it rises and falls. Feel the sensation of air hitting your nostrils.

3. Notice any physical sensations you experience. Do you feel pain? Tightness? Buzzing? Warmth? Cold? Openness? Constriction? Physical symptoms of an illness?

4. Ask your body what it's trying to communicate to you. If something in your body is here to help you get your needs met, protect you, or get through to you about something in your life that might be out of alignment, what is the message it wants you to hear? Invite your Inner Pilot Light to answer. Listen to the wisdom of what comes up.

5. Now open your eyes and let your physical symptom or illness write you a letter. For example, if you have back pain, let your back pain write to you. (Dear You, . . . Love, Your Back Pain.) If you have cancer, let your cancer pen the letter. (Dear You, . . . Love, Your Cancer.)

6. Write a response. Once your physical symptom or illness has written to you, write back. (Dear Back Pain, . . . Love, Me.)

7. Let the back-and-forth dialogue ensue as long as you're learning from your body. Take notice of what comes up in the letters. This is your Inner Pilot Light speaking through your body. Listen up.

8. Thank your body for its wisdom. Promise to keep in touch more often.

Often, we choose to ignore the messages sent to us from our Inner Pilot Lights via the body, either because we're not listening or because we don't like what the messages have to say. Tapping into this body wisdom may command change, and we may not be fond of hearing those messages if we're understandably scared and not yet ready to change.

For example, a nagging cough may be your body's way of telling you it's time to quit smoking, but if you're not willing to quit, you'll likely distance yourself from your Inner Pilot Light or ignore your body. A lump in your neck may tell you it's time to go to the doctor, but if you're afraid of what you might hear, you may ignore it until the lump becomes so great that you lose your voice. Pain during sex may be your body's way of saying it no longer feels safe in your relationship and it's time to move on. Cancer may be telling you to stop over-caretaking everyone else and start caring for yourself. A heart attack may be telling you to slow down and relax your workaholic, type A tendencies.

If you let them, physical symptoms can build a bridge between you and your Inner Pilot Light. When you learn to listen to the nuances of what your Inner Pilot Light is telling you, the body may no longer have to manifest these messages physically, and you may prevent physical symptoms or serious disease. But if you're not skilled at hearing this internal voice, your body can be your guide. Within your body lies the perfect compass that will guide you back home, if only you listen. For more tips on tapping into the wisdom of your Inner Pilot Light, sign up for inspiring daily messages at InnerPilotLight.com or read my book *The Daily Flame*.

The next exercise is modified from the Internal Family Systems (IFS) model, created by family therapist Richard Schwartz, Ph.D., which we discussed earlier. In the IFS model, we are all a multiplicity of parts, and some of our parts may use the body to get our attention so we can heal the wounded parts they protect. The following exercise may help reveal to you why you may have parts that are using your body to help you get the healing you need.

Diagnostic Exercise #2: Communicate with Your Symptom or Illness as a "Part," Using IFS

1. Go inside and put your attention on the part of the body that is troubling you. Ask if there is a part that is using your body to get your attention right now. Focus your attention there.

2. Get to know this part. Can you visualize it? Does it have a color, shape, or image? Does it say anything or evoke a feeling? Can you get close to it? If so, what happens to it?

3. Notice how you feel toward this part. Are you feeling any of the "8 Cs of Self"—curious, calm, compassionate, clear, courageous, connected, confident, and creative? Or do you have other parts that don't like this part, parts that might be scared, angry, or repulsed perhaps. If you're feeling anything but the 8Cs, ask if other parts will relax and step aside and let you get to know the part that might be causing problems in the body. If they won't relax, you might need to consult an IFS therapist.

4. Befriend the part. See if it will let you get close. Let it know you're curious why it might be using the body to get your attention. See if you can figure out how it thinks it's protecting you. What does it want you to know? How did it get its job? What is it afraid would happen if it quit doing its job? If it didn't have to do this job, what else would it like to do? How old is this part? How old does it think you are? Is there anything else it would like you to know?

5. The part may reveal an "exile" it is protecting, who is often a young inner child who may feel scared, ashamed, worthless, unlovable, sad, discarded, or other feelings that may be hard to bear. If this happens, you may want to get professional help with an IFS therapist or someone else who specializes in cutting-edge trauma therapies. Tending to the parts that use the body to avoid feeling these painful emotions, and healing the parts that carry those emotional burdens may allow the body to heal in remarkable ways.

Work/Life Balance

Although true work/life balance is almost impossible—many believe it's merely a crazy-making myth that leaves us striving for perfection and feeling chronically inadequate—it's important to be mindful of how we spend our time and whether we're prioritizing activities that induce the relaxation response. While finding the perfect balance between work life, family life, and personal life is challenging, and while I don't think it's always possible to have a balanced day, I do think it's possible to have a balanced week. I make a practice of switching out the radical self-care practices I wish I could do daily but don't always manage to fit in. For example, in a perfect world, my average day would start with waking up and meditating, practicing yoga, making a homemade batch of green juice, and preparing a healthy, organic breakfast to enjoy with my family. Then I'd write, paint, attend to other work matters, have lunch with a friend, work some more, go for a hike, read to my daughter, cook another healthy meal for dinner, and end my day enjoying hot sex with my partner.

As if!

The reality is that some days I'm on a tight deadline and I work a 14-hour day, barely seeing my partner or my daughter, skipping my meditation and hike, eating takeout, overlooking my creative pursuits, and barely managing to kiss my partner goodnight, much less rally for a little nookie. But I try to make that a rare occasion. And I try to balance it out. If I have a day like that on Monday,

I do everything within my power to prioritize my family and my self-care on Tuesday, even if it means my work is delayed. By Wednesday, I look back over the week to see whether I've gotten in my meditation, exercised, eaten well, loved on my honey, spent quality time with my daughter, and allowed myself to create, all of which induce relaxation responses in me, nurture my mind and body, and keep me happy and healthy. By the end of the week, hopefully I've had a balanced week, even if I never got around to accomplishing all the work and self-care habits I aim to include as a regular part of my life.

The next exercise is designed to help you assess your work/life balance so you can get a feel for whether imbalances in your Whole Health Cairn may be harming your health. Pay attention to which stones in your Whole Health Cairn induce relaxation responses for you and which ones are stressors.

Diagnostic Exercise #3: How Balanced Is Your Whole Health Cairn?

1. Photocopy seven copies of the Whole Health Cairn from this book (page 87) or print out copies you can download at MindOverMedicineBook.com.

2. Each day of the week, using crayons or markers, color in the stones in the Whole Health Cairn that you nurtured. For example, if you meditated, fill in your Spirituality stone. If you had good sex, fill in Sexuality. If you took good care of your physical body, fill in Physical Health. If you took time out to be a good mom or nurtured a relationship with your best friend, fill in your Relationships stone. If all you did was work, fill in your Work/Life Purpose stone . . . and so forth.

3. At the end of the week, pay attention to where you are focusing most of your time and energy. Are you skipping the same stones every day? Is your Whole Health Cairn out of balance? Which stones need attention?

A Practice of Inquiry for Self-Diagnosis

The next exercise is designed to help you use the Whole Health Cairn as a diagnostic tool to identify aspects of your life that might be triggering your stress responses and predisposing you to illness. In other words, where is each stone in the Whole Health Cairn on the spectrum of medicine versus poison? It's also designed to help you get a feel for what activities in your life might elicit the relaxation response as part of your treatment. The goal of this exercise is to help you identify issues that are getting between you and optimal health.

Of all the practices in this six-step process, this one exercise is the most vital. It can also be the hardest. So please listen to your Inner Pilot Light as you work through this section. And call upon your support system. If you can go through this exercise with a therapist or Whole Health Medicine Institute graduate, even better.

Diagnostic Exercise #4: Make the Diagnosis for Yourself

Part One

Ask yourself this series of questions, and be sure you go at your own speed. Take as much time as you need to answer the questions fully and honestly. And if you need to take a break or even stop, that's okay too. I can assure you that if you're willing to be truthful with yourself in answering the questions in this section, your Inner Pilot Light will grant you a precious gift—the opportunity to know what's true for you so you can gain healing insight and make The Diagnosis for yourself.

You may want to talk through these questions out loud, by yourself or with a loved one. Or you may want to journal about them. To download The Diagnosis Journal, which leaves you room to write in the answers to the following questions, visit MindOver MedicineBook.com.

Try to stay grounded, embodied, and present as you do this exercise. Also, be infinitely compassionate with yourself during this process. If you find yourself spiraling downward into negative thoughts, take a break, get support, and come back to it later with the help of your support system. Make sure to be radically nurturing with yourself. As you answer these questions, focus on gratitude for the blessings in your life, fill your life with pleasure, and be your own best friend. Doing so can ease the discomfort you may feel and keep you focusing on what's working in your life so you can be fearless enough to face and change what isn't.

INNER PILOT LIGHT

- Am I living an authentic life aligned with all that I yearn for deep in my heart?

- Do I make an effort to have my heart's longings met?

- What does my Inner Pilot Light want me to know?

- When my intuition communicates with me, how much do I listen?

- What truth am I unwilling to face in my life right now?

- What within me am I holding back? What longs to be set free?

- What comes between me and my Inner Pilot Light?

- Am I willing to risk everything in order to listen to my Inner Pilot Light? If not, why not?

- Do I trust that I have an Inner Pilot Light?

- Do I trust that it's safe to follow my Inner Pilot Light's guidance?

- Do I have ways of discerning whether voices in my head are my Inner Pilot Light or other parts that are trying to push an agenda?

- Who would I be if I were fearless?

- On a scale of one to ten, how much do I love and accept myself, even the parts of me I demonize or other people demonize?

RELATIONSHIPS

- How do I feel about my romantic life?
- How do I feel about my friends and support network?
- What are the repetitive relationship patterns that continue to appear in my life?
- Is there someone I need to forgive? Am I willing to forgive this person? Why or why not?
- Am I getting my natural human need for love, attention, nurturing, and belonging adequately met?
- How vulnerable am I willing to be with the people in my life?
- If my loved ones were to die—or have already died— how much have I left unsaid?
- In the context of my relationships, is there always somebody wrong and somebody right?
- Do I tend to be the narcissist or the codependent in any relationships that may be symbiotic?
- Do I ask for help when I need it? Am I more comfortable giving or receiving?
- How often do I feel used in my relationships? Am I willing to release the victim or savior role in order to heal?
- Do I feel worthy of love and affection?
- What would I change about the love in my life if I had a magic wand?
- Do I need professional help to deal with one or more of the relationships in my life? If so, will the person I need help with come with me to therapy, or will I need to do this alone?

WORK/LIFE PURPOSE

- What does my Inner Pilot Light want me to know about my work?

- What are my natural gifts, the things everyone knows I'm good at?

- Is how I spend most of my day in line with my talents and purpose?

- Does my work feed my need to be a beacon of love and make the world a better place?

- How does my body feel when I'm at work? How does my mind feel when I'm at work?

- Is my work a job, a career, a calling, or a mixture of the three?

- Do I feel like my work is a calling at least 40 percent of the time?

- In what area of my life have I been to hell and back? Might I serve those still in hell in this area?

- If someone handed me a microphone and put me in front of an audience on the last day of my life, what would I say to the world?

- If all my financial needs were met and the needs of my family were met, what would I do with my time?

- If I took fear out of the equation, what would I change about how I spend my days?

- Is my job the bridge to getting me where I want to go?

- Am I learning valuable things in my day job that I'm supposed to know, even if I don't love the work I do?

- Is my work life impacting my health?

CREATIVITY

- What lights my creative fire? Who or what is my muse?
- Am I clear on what my soul wants to create?
- What helps my creativity flow freely?
- What kinds of creative projects light me up? Am I doing these things regularly?
- What creative projects did I engage in as a child?
- If I had all the time and money in the world, what would I create?
- How do I feel when I don't feel inspired?
- Is my inner critic interfering with my creative process?
- Am I afraid to risk failure?
- Am I willing to be with the frustration of the creative process?
- Do I feel worthy of expressing myself creatively?
- What does my family believe about creativity?

SPIRITUALITY

- What makes me feel spiritually connected?
- What do I consider sacred?
- Is it time to start a daily meditation practice?
- Are there other spiritual practices that would benefit me?
- Am I free to be authentic in my spiritual life?
- If I don't consider myself "religious" or even believe in a Higher Power, am I finding other ways to nurture my spiritual self?
- What are my thoughts and feelings about religion? What negative thoughts do I have about spirituality or religion?

- Do I have spiritual traumas that need to be treated?

- What does my family believe about spirituality?

- Are there ways in which I use my spirituality or religion to judge others?

- Am I worthy of experiencing a deep connection with the Divine?

- Would joining the right spiritual community elicit relaxation responses in my body?

SEXUALITY

- What do I truly desire sexually? Am I fulfilling that desire?

- What will help support my authentic sexual self?

- What fears, beliefs, or hang-ups keep me from being as sexually honest and openly expressed as I might wish to be?

- How do I feel about my first sexual experience?

- What from my sexual past or present life may be in need of healing?

- What *really* turns me on? What *really* turns me off?

- How do I feel about having sex when I don't want to?

- Do I feel sensual when I'm not having sex?

- What does my family believe about sexuality?

- If I could do anything sexually and nobody else ever had to know, what would I do?

MONEY

- What are my thoughts and feelings about my financial situation?

- How financially healthy am I?

- How do I define financial health, success, or abundance?
- How much wealth would be "enough"?
- What does my family believe about money?
- What limiting beliefs about my finances do I need to release?
- Do I have enough money to support me in case of an emergency?
- Is it possible to be poor and happy?
- How much time do I spend thinking about money?
- What negative stories do you tell yourself about what it would be like to be wealthy? Might some of these stories be blocking financial security?

ENVIRONMENT

- Am I living where my Inner Pilot Light wants to live?
- When I look around at my surroundings, do I love what I see?
- Am I surrounded by beauty? Does my environment include nature?
- How healthy is my environment?
- What environmental exposures might be affecting my health?
- On a scale of one to ten, how "green" am I?
- What efforts do I make to reduce the toxic load on my body caused by my environment?
- How might I eliminate unnecessary clutter from my environment?
- Do I feel worthy of living in a healing, peaceful environment I love?

MENTAL HEALTH

- What are the painful patterns that keep repeating themselves in my life?
- Am I depressed or anxious on a regular basis?
- Do traumas from my past still cause me suffering?
- Do I need to start seeing a therapist to treat life's inevitable traumas?
- Is my trauma history impacting my physical body?
- Do I need treatment for an addiction?
- On a scale of one to ten, what is my quality of life?
- Do I feel worthy of being happy?
- Do I tend to see the glass half full or half empty?
- How much time do I spend engaging in negative conversations such as unkind gossip, criticism of another person, or complaining?
- Do I express gratitude for what I appreciate in my life on a regular basis?
- Do I get caught up in what I lack rather than appreciating what I have?

PHYSICAL HEALTH

- How are my diet and exercise habits?
- How compliant am I with my health-care provider's recommendations and protocols?
- What unhealthy habits do I need to release?
- How are my energy levels?
- How many hours of sleep am I getting?
- Are there supplements I might benefit from taking?
- Am I optimizing using food as medicine?

- Would adding green juice as a supplement or cleanse benefit me?

- Am I willing to invest time, money, and energy in taking better care of my body?

- Do I treat my body as a temple for my soul?

- How do I feel about aging?

WRAP-UP

- How much am I willing to fully accept myself in all my divine imperfections?

- How much permission do I give myself to make mistakes?

- Am I willing to fiercely love and accept myself during my healing journey?

- Do I feel I have everything I need in order to make my body ripe for miracles?

- Am I willing to use what I've learned to write The Prescription for myself and make changes in my life?

Part Two

Using the answers to these questions, can you identify the root causes associated with your illness? Are there any issues in your Whole Health Cairn that might be triggering your stress responses and harming your body? Are there activities that would elicit relaxation responses in your body that you're not utilizing? Have these questions helped illuminate any blind spots in your life you needed to see in order to be optimally healthy? How could you transform each stone in the Whole Health Cairn into medicine, not poison?

Within each category, take notes in The Diagnosis Journal, which you can download at MindOverMedicineBook.com, anything you've identified that you intuit might be interfering with your optimal health.

Congratulations! You just made The Diagnosis.

Step Five: Write The Prescription for Yourself

Now it's time to make a whole-health treatment plan of radical self-care.

When you get sick, your doctor may prescribe a different kind of treatment plan. For example, if you get cancer and you have a smart, savvy, holistic physician, your treatment plan may include surgery, chemotherapy, a nourishing raw-food or vegan diet, a host of supplements meant to ramp up your immune system, a support group to help you deal with the emotions of cancer, and a yoga practice to keep you centered.

That kind of treatment plan will get you far. But if the root cause of your weakened immune system is loneliness, job stress, a toxic relationship, or untreated trauma, treating the cancer without treating the root causes may help in the short term, but it may not be permanent. The cancer may come back—or you'll wind up with some other illness. In order to optimally prevent and treat disease so you don't keep circling back to a weakened, sick body, you must, must, *must* address the root causes that make you susceptible to illness in the first place, while listening to your Inner Pilot Light and letting it help you choose how to maximize what conventional medicine has to offer in a way that is in alignment for you.

That's what writing The Prescription is all about. Your Prescription may include conventional medical treatments, but it won't stop there. It will also include whatever is needed in order to treat the problem areas you identified in Step Four.

Part of writing The Prescription for yourself is stepping up to the plate as the head honcho of your health care. Remember, you're the boss. Everyone else is in service to you. Your doctor might be able to prescribe your pills, but only *you* can write The Prescription for how your life needs to change in order to optimize your whole health. Your Prescription is the intuitively guided, whole health action plan for how you're planning to treat your condition, which may be as simple as one right next step, or it may be a three-page document of action steps you intend to take to treat every misalignment in every stone of the Whole Health Cairn.

Here's how you can get started.

A Therapeutic Exercise: Write the Prescription for Yourself

1.   Grab a pen and pull out a few sheets of paper or your journal, or download The Prescription form from MindOverMedicineBook.com.

2.   Pull out The Diagnosis you've created for yourself on sheets of paper, in your journal, or in The Diagnosis Journal you downloaded.

3.   Take a moment to close your eyes and tap into the healing wisdom of your Inner Pilot Light. Remind yourself to stay open, loving, and compassionate with yourself. When you feel centered, relaxed, and intuitively open, open your eyes.

4.   Ask yourself, "What do I need in order to heal? What will it take to live a life my body will love?" Tune into your body and see if your body itself gives you any clues. Stay in silence and listen deeply.

5.   You might only get one action item, which is fine. Or you might feel guided to go through each of the items you listed in The Diagnosis, ask yourself what you can do to take action in order to treat any root cause of illness you've identified. Trust your intuition and try not to judge what comes up. Remember, you don't have to actually implement these action steps yet, but you do have to be honest with yourself. Don't censor anything. *Nobody ever has to read this but you.*

6.   If you've identified an issue but aren't sure how to heal it, check out my blog at LissaRankin.com, where I write about a variety of healing practices related to every stone in the Whole Health Cairn.

When I first started teaching the Six Steps to Healing Yourself to patients outside my medical practice, particularly when I was teaching Mind Over Medicine workshops to groups, I bumped into a curious phenomenon. After people completed Step Five, I would say, "Of course there are no guarantees in the real world, but if we lived in a magical universe where you had a 100 percent guarantee that if you followed through on every single item in your Prescription, you'd be cured, how many of you would do it?" Time and time again, I was shocked to discover that only about half of the people raised their hands. When this happened the first time, I said, "Those of you who didn't raise your hands, please stand up. I want to talk to you!"

When they stood up, looking sheepish, I said, "Don't worry. I'm not going to shame you. I just want to understand why you wouldn't do what you wrote down."

Looking at the floor, one woman said, "I know I need to leave my loveless marriage, but I'm too afraid. He pays all the bills and we have a prenup. How would I pay for the lifestyle I live?"

Another looked up at the ceiling when he said, "But I'm getting a disability check, and I hated my old job. If I got cured, I'd have to go back." One by one, each person who stood up spoke to their resistance.

"I used to caretake my aging parents, who were abusive to me when I was young. Now that I'm sick, I don't have to do that, but if I got better, my brother would fire the nurse and expect me to do it, since I'm the one who lives close to her. I'd rather die than go back to taking care of my parents."

"This sounds lame, but if I'm honest with myself, being sick is my excuse for not following through on my promise—to myself and my loved ones—to finally write the book I've been saying I'd write someday. I realize I'm more afraid of failure than I am of being sick."

"I know I'm selling my soul in my job, and I hate it, but I'm not qualified to do anything else."

"I just know this illness is related to my childhood sexual abuse, but honestly, I'm just not ready to face that demon head-on."

I was stunned. Until that point, I hadn't realized that back when I was practicing medicine and applying these six steps with patients, part of what I was doing during the hour I had with my patients during each visit was helping them address and treat their resistance to making the sometimes dramatic life changes they knew they needed to make. Even then, they were often frightened to take the risks their Prescriptions invited them to take. This is why I wrote *The Fear Cure* as the follow-up to *Mind Over Medicine*. I realized that if fear was driving someone's decision making, the stress response evoked by the fear would make them sick and prevent full recovery. Fear would also prevent them from doing what they knew intuitively they needed to do in order to make their bodies ripe for miracles.

This epiphany changed how I work with the Six Steps and made it obvious that addressing fear and resistance head on was fundamental to this process. Without treating the fear and resistance, at least half of people would fail to follow through on what they intuitively knew they needed to do in order to optimize their chance for radical remission. That awareness led me to add a sixth step that didn't exist in the original edition of *Mind Over Medicine.*

STEP SIX: Treat Your Fears and Resistance

In order for the Six Steps to Healing Yourself to truly optimize your health, you'll need to be honest with yourself about your fears and resistance, do what you must in order to address your fears, and creatively problem solve how to get your needs met so you don't unconsciously sabotage this process by relying on your illness to get core needs met.

It's natural to have resistance to change. We all have it. Even positive change can evoke fear and resistance. But unless you lean into the fear and resistance, become intimate with it as if it's an IFS part, negotiate with it, and get creative about how to deal with it, your fears and resistance might convince you to change nothing in your life. And if you change nothing, it's unlikely that your health will improve.

How can you get creative about dealing with fear and resistance? For example, let's say you intuit that unhealed trauma is impacting your health, but you're frightened of seeing a trauma therapist because you're afraid you'll get so flooded by painful feelings and memories that you won't able to function. In this case, you might ask a trusted friend to come to your first therapy session with you so you won't feel so terrified, and you might need your therapist to help you deal with the fear of getting flooded before anything else happens in therapy.

Or maybe you're afraid of ending a marriage or quitting a job because doing so will interrupt your financial security. This may be a valid concern. You might have to downsize, liquidate some of your assets, move in with a family member while you get back on your feet, or even borrow money for a while. If you're getting a disability check from a job you hated, you may need to be willing to give up that disability check and find a job you love instead.

You may be consciously aware of some but not all of your fear and resistance. For most people, the fear and resistance you're conscious of are like the tip of an iceberg, with even more buried in the subconscious. Below the level of your conscious awareness, you may even have parts that don't want to keep living. Especially if you've had a hard life and your quality of life has been poor, it would be understandable that parts of you might think it's time to check out. Not that you're having suicidal thoughts or consciously aware of this impulse, but the waning will to live may be running the show from under the surface of your conscious awareness. Such unconscious interference can dramatically influence your healing journey if left untreated.

Remember that the parts that are scared or resistant are only parts, not your whole self. You probably have other parts that are very enthusiastic, even excited about making these changes and optimizing your health. These parts may be polarized against each other, stuck in an inner war. But you don't have to choose sides. Your job is to love and accept all of these parts, without blending with them or letting them drive your choices and actions.

Keep in mind that these parts can get pretty noisy inside your head, since they sincerely think they're protecting you, even if they're obviously sabotaging efforts to heal. It doesn't help to bully these parts. Bullying them only makes them more scared and resistant. If your Inner Pilot Light earns the trust of these scared and resistant parts, over time, those parts will let your Inner Pilot Light take the lead when it comes to decision-making and action steps.

Not sure if you have resistance? Try this exercise.

Exercise: Identify Your Fears & Resistance

- Close your eyes and turn your attention inward. Breathe deeply and center yourself.

- With compassionate curiosity, ask any fearful parts or resistant parts to make themselves known. Let them know you understand that they're simply trying to protect you. Make sure those parts understand that you're not going to bully them or shame them. You just want to become intimate with them and help them relax. See if those parts will reveal themselves to you. If they do, simply turn your attention to them without judging them. Let them unveil themselves so you understand why some parts might not want you to do what your intuition has guided you to do in order to get well. Be aware that some parts might not want you to get well at all, not because they're intentionally trying to sabotage your healing journey, but because they think they're protecting you.

- If those parts are willing, ask them what they're afraid would happen if they stopped doing their job to protect you through fear or resistance. Listen generously to discover what they might reveal. Remind your parts that you won't pressure them to do anything they're not ready to do.

- You may need to earn the trust of these parts by showing up in daily meditations to let them see that you have an Inner Pilot Light, which can be trusted to make good decisions that benefit all of your parts. Keep showing up every day to check on your parts. Over time and with experience, your scared and resistant parts are likely to quiet down and let you do what you must. Once you discover the wounded parts they may be protecting, you may need to see a therapist to help "unburden" these parts so your scared or resistant parts will stop sabotaging your healing journey.

242

Note: To become more intimate with these parts and begin to heal them, consider listening to Richard Schwartz's Sounds True audio program Greater Than the Sum of Our Parts: Discovering Your True Self Through Internal Family Systems Therapy. *For more in-depth healing work, or if your scared, resistant parts continue to drive your decisions and actions, consider working with a skilled IFS therapist.*

You could make a valid argument that fear and resistance should be treated as Step One to make the whole process easier from the get-go. In fact, in healing modalities such as Advanced Integrative Therapy (AIT), treating such resistance is built into the model right at the beginning of therapy, in order to hasten the process and limit blocks that might interfere with healing. Others might argue that Step Two (spiritual surrender) should come before Step One (belief), and they would have a valid point too. As I've come to realize, these steps are not entirely linear. While they're presented in a linear fashion in this book, you'll discover as you come to work with the Six Steps to Healing Yourself that you may experience stepping forward and then stepping back, in and out of these steps. Do not be concerned if you notice yourself doing this. Engage with this process however it feels most natural to you.

You may weave in and out of feeling empowered and feeling victimized. You may experience rapid expansion into awareness, growth, and insight, only to notice that fear, resistance, and self-sabotage have hijacked your efforts at self-healing. You may wholeheartedly commit to a practice of spiritual surrender, only to realize that you're back to your old ways of longing for greater ease, grasping for what you desire, attaching to outcomes, and trying to control life. The key is to be gentle with yourself. Don't judge yourself or shame yourself. Just notice what's happening, and just as you would do in a meditation practice, keep coming back to the Six Step practice, over and over. This is a practice you will most likely never fully master, and that is just fine. There's a reason we call it a "practice"!

In fact, just to show you how fluid the order of the steps may be, let me suggest revisiting Step Two at the end of our journey here, just in case it's helpful.

Surrender Again

As you've worked these six steps, you may have started attaching to outcomes again, making a story that you've done everything right and therefore you deserve a permanent cure. If your disease fails to resolve, you may even blame yourself or judge yourself for somehow not doing it right. Remember, you participate in the co-creative process, but you are not in control. Go back to the God Box meditation and repeat the practice every time you find yourself grasping for cure with a desperation that will reactivate stress responses. Make it a practice to keep holding the paradox of being proactive to optimize your health while also letting go of attachment to outcomes and repeating the simple prayer, "Let us pray for that which is most right." Every time you backslide or find yourself disappointed, scared, or trying to control life, let go. Over time, the practice gets easier. If you need support from others who are practicing the Six Steps, join us online at HealingSoulTribe.com or find out the status of our live groups at HealAtLast.org.

Take Baby Steps

Once you've completed the six steps, it helps to start small. Just pick one small action step from your Prescription, something you feel ready to do. All you need to know is your next right step. Hang your Prescription somewhere you can see it often. Once you've implemented the first step, glance at your Prescription every day and wait until the next right step reveals itself to you. Manage your expectations for yourself appropriately, knowing that you're not likely to implement every single action item in the first week. It may take weeks or months or years even—and that's okay.

What if you're not willing to take action to make changes that will help you live a life your body will love? What if you know what it will take to get well and you just can't take the leap of faith? If that's the case, be kind to yourself. You can't rush your healing. Maybe it's not time yet. Remember, you'll know when it's time to take a leap of faith when the pain of staying put exceeds the fear of the unknown. If you're not there yet, it's okay to wait.

Once you know what needs to change in your life and you decide you're going to go for it, be exceedingly compassionate with yourself. Go easy. Take baby steps. Reward yourself often. Serve yourself a heaping helping of acceptance, gratitude, and love. Give yourself permission to overdose on pleasure, love, beauty, comfort, and anything else you'll need in order to make yourself ready to do what you must. You'll need it to fuel your journey. Dousing yourself with self-care fertilizes the ground for the transformation that awaits you. As the saying often attributed to Anaïs Nin goes, "And the day came when the risk to remain tight in a bud was more painful than the risk it took to blossom." Your day to blossom will come, and if it's aligned for your greatest good, it's possible, but not guaranteed, that cure will follow.

Keep in mind that it's hard to anticipate how you will feel about your self-healing journey, so I want to give you a little heads-up. Having supported the self-healing journeys of many people, I can attest to the fact that the journey is different for everyone, and outcomes vary. Surprisingly, some people have an unexpected response to a good outcome. For example, one of my patients had been suffering from a chronic illness for 20 years when we started working through this process together. After three months of regular sessions and intense work on her part, her disease vanished. I was thrilled! It worked!

But she was grief stricken, barely able to get out of bed every morning, even though her physical symptoms were completely gone. Mourning the 20 years she felt she had lost from a disease she now realized she could have cured solely with the power of her consciousness and lifestyle changes, she spun into depression until a daily gratitude practice, an opportunity to serve those less fortunate than her, and the birth of her grandson pulled her out of her despair. Her experience helped me realize how important it is to live in the present when you're going through a process like this. Remaining optimistic, focusing on gratitude, and appreciating what you have is vital to keep you from spinning into regrets and sadness about what might have been. If you're blessed to experience a radical remission as the result of this process, it's okay to mourn the years of suffering and feel the regret fully, but do try to find your gratitude as well.

Remember, you were blessed with a second chance, and you have an opportunity to take what you've learned and use it to help others.

Another patient of mine who experienced radical remission had the complete opposite experience. Although she too had suffered from her illness, she never once looked back when her illness was cured. She viewed her cure as a miracle that opened her up to a richer spiritual life and transformed not just her health but her romantic life, her professional life, and where she lived. She used her story to inspire others and now sees her journey through illness as the wake-up call that served as the catalyst for her spiritual growth.

Yet another patient worked through this whole process with such courage, even in the face of rapidly declining health. She fearlessly faced her truth; healed a lot of unresolved trauma, realigned all sorts of relationship contracts in her life; started living her dream; released old resentments; let go of old, stale negative core beliefs; forgave people she had been holding grudges against since childhood; and aligned with her Inner Pilot Light in every aspect of her life. Although she ultimately succumbed to her illness, she did so with such grace that her death was a healing to dozens of other people, especially her family. She wasn't cured, but she died healed. Hundreds showed up for her funeral to express their gratitude for a life well lived and well ended.

What more can we hope for as we navigate this journey? It's a win-win situation. Whether or not you're cured, you will be healed, and your healing may offer a healing to others.

I encourage you to remember that it will be a rebirth, if you're open to experiencing it, and on the other side, you will expand in ways you may not even be able to imagine. Circling back around and surrendering attachment to outcomes when you're sick, after you've done everything within your power to make your body ripe for miracles, allows illness to be an opportunity for spiritual awakening. If you let it, being sick can show you the trailheads where your greatest healing lies, light a fire under you to reprioritize your life, remind you to appreciate what you have, allow you to align your life with your Inner Pilot Light, give you the courage to live in the moment, and bring you closer to loved ones and to the Divine.

When I did an art project I called "The Woman Inside Project," during which I cast the torsos of women with breast cancer using medical-grade plaster, while interviewing them about the beauty that lies within them, almost every woman whose body I sculpted said cancer was the best thing that ever happened to her because it led her to take steps in her life that turned out to effect lasting positive change.

We shouldn't have to wait for illness to realign with our truth, but often we do. Just like I needed my Perfect Storm to wake up, many need to get sick so they get jolted out of their complacency and start living as if they might die tomorrow. If illness strikes, it's a potent opportunity to wake up, even if part of what we're here to learn and teach is how to die with grace. While I believe miracles are always possible, sometimes a cure simply doesn't happen. We must make peace with this fact. If you set upon a quest to heal yourself while attaching to the outcome of complete cure, and then you find yourself still sick, you may wind up pitched into the despair of the dark night of the soul. But if you start with the prayer "Let us do that which is most right," then do everything within your power to make your body ripe for miracles—and *then you let go and trust the journey*—you pave the way for peace, serenity, and joy beyond your wildest imagining.

For Practitioners & Caregivers: Discerning Good Candidates for the Six Steps to Healing Yourself

The Six Steps to Healing Yourself are not for everyone, so if you're a health-care professional, therapist, healer, or caregiver, let's talk about how to discern good candidates for this healing method and how to deal with those who aren't. The stark truth is that not everyone is ready to approach a life-threatening or chronic illness in this way, and that's okay. The professionals I train in the Whole Health Medicine Institute often ask me how we can convert patients who may not seem like good candidates into people who are open-minded, curious, disciplined, motivated, spiritually aware, and committed to doing whatever it takes to optimize health outcomes using mental, emotional, and spiritual healing medicines. I tell them, "Everyone is entitled to their own journey." All we can do is gently make the invitation without burdening patients with our own agendas. As a practitioner or a caregiver for someone who is sick, you can try giving patients a copy of this book or Kelly Turner's *Radical Remission*. You can be, as Richard Schwartz describes it, "a merchant of hope for hopeless parts." But ultimately, just as pressuring an addict to quit usually backfires, badgering someone who is sick and trying to convert them to your point of view will only alienate someone you care about.

Your well-intended invitation is most likely to be warmly received if you have zero attachment to someone's yes or no. If you approach a resistant person with a missionary's zeal and a dogmatic sense that your way is better than their way, you're likely to alienate a person who really needs your unconditional love and support. If you really want to be helpful, put your own agenda aside and ask with an open heart what they really need. Trust that they know what's best for them better than you do, even if that means they may stay sick or even die from their condition. Keep in mind that this might still be the outcome, even if they do everything you would do were you in the same situation.

Everyone is entitled to their own journey. If this upsets you, treat the parts of yourself that are frightened of losing someone you love, the parts that are afraid of failing to cure someone, or the parts who think they have any business micromanaging and controlling other people's lives.

In my own practice, I found that some patients, especially older patients who were raised with a more heavy-handed, patriarchal model of medicine, felt inadequate, inexperienced and insecure about participating in their own treatment plan. They would wave a dismissive hand at me and say, "Oh, I wouldn't know anything about such things. That's why I go to doctors." Some felt frightened of what they might uncover and trembled at the idea that there might be dragons under the veils of their denial. Many sheepishly admitted to being content giving their power away to doctors who would just tell them what to do and relieve them of taking any responsibility for their health outcome.

Some patients I determined as poor candidates for this type of healing work, and over time, I learned to trust my intuition about who might benefit from this Six Step process and who might not. My assessment of who would benefit most from this work was consistent with the findings of a study done by psychologist, scientist, researcher, and cancer survivor Alistair Cunningham, Ph.D., at the University of Toronto. He and his team published an article "Fighting for life: A qualitative analysis of the process of psychotherapy-assisted self-help in patients with metastatic cancer."[4] Patients with metastatic cancer were treated with group therapy and assessed for a variety of psycho-spiritual factors that might influence survival. Both length of survival and quality of life were tracked in individuals with equally unfavorable medical prognoses. The researchers found these factors to be associated with longer survival and higher quality of life:

- Sufficient flexibility and dedication to make an active response to the diagnosis
- Changes in habit of thought and activity
- Relaxation practices and meditation
- Mental imaging
- Cognitive monitoring and questioning beliefs
- Becoming involved in a search for meaning in one's life

So what led to poor survival and lower quality of life?

- Inflexibility associated with low self-esteem or fixed worldview that the subject saw no reason to alter
- Skepticism about the potential impact of psychological self-help techniques or one's ability to apply them
- Other activities seemed more important or immediately appealing
- Meaning was habitually sought outside the person, rather than through internal searching

- Strong, contrary views about the validity of spiritual ideas
- Need for control so strong that recommended changes were rejected

The conclusions of studies such as this, which attempt to draw causal links between psychotherapy and improved cancer outcomes, are mixed, most likely because there is no standardization between studies regarding the kind of therapy, and not all therapies are created equal. However, studies such as Cunningham's trend toward what the patients, doctors, therapists, and CAM providers I've worked with observe. At least anecdotally, health outliers universally seem to be characterized by the first list of qualities. While such traits are not an automatic recipe for cure, they do seem to increase the chances of becoming someone who is primed to experience radical remission.

As you work with this material, in your own life or with loved ones or clients, it's important to keep in mind that this kind of work can be painful. It's understandable why some people just aren't ready to touch the pain they may encounter on a healing journey like this. Our culture's tendency to try to avoid pain at all costs is part of the epidemic of mental and physical illness so many people face. We have to remember that it hurts to be human, and as much as conventional medicine tries to sell a story that a pill can take away all of your pain, it's a lie. Pain is part of being in a human body, and there's simply no way to get away from it. In fact, pain always arrives for a good reason. It's our body's or our heart's way of saying, "Pay Attention Inside Now (PAIN)." When pain arrives, something needs to be felt, moved through, and healed. When we try to bypass or numb pain, it backfires.

Have compassion for yourself or others if you determine that you're not ready for this process. A seed will have been planted and maybe someday, you'll be ready. If you've read this far, the seeds will bloom if and when the time is right.

Maybe now is the time. If you're on the cusp of transformation and ready to face the truth about yourself, your life, and your illness, you'll have the opportunity to awaken to the calm, grounded, joyful fulfillment that comes with living in alignment with your Inner Pilot Light. And when you do, you relax your body, flip on your self-repair mechanisms, and make the body ripe for miracles. Remember, when you enter into uncertainty and you don't know what the future holds, *anything is possible.*

When You're Healed but Not Cured

Keep in mind that healing and curing are not the same thing. I know. I witnessed it in my father.

When my father got sick with a brain tumor that wound up being metastatic melanoma, Dad believed he would beat it. He was young—too young—and he was an optimist with great faith, a supportive community, a family that adored him, and a wide-open heart. Dad certainly didn't do anything wrong to earn his cancer. He was a wonderful man who led a blessed life.

But he died anyway. It felt so unfair.

He died like a master. He called all his loved ones to his bedside so he could ask our permission to transition. He told us he had no regrets, no love unexpressed, no dream unlived, no song unsung. He felt his mission on earth was complete and he wanted us to bless his decision to cross over. We didn't understand. He was very functional still, with all his faculties still intact even though he had a massive brain tumor. What was his plan? Physician-assisted suicide?

No, he said. He planned to simply go to sleep and die. That night he asked us to prepare his last meal and he offered each of us a blessing. Then he kissed us goodnight, went to sleep, and never woke up. Within twenty-four hours, he breathed his last breath. We were shocked and in awe. As a doctor, I've witnessed a lot of deaths, but none more beautiful than my father's. Dad was healed but not cured, and this might happen to you or someone you love too.

Some Are Both Healed and Cured

It's also entirely possible that you could have a radical remission. You could be like the 77-year-old man reported in this case study in the medical literature.[5] He was diagnosed with pancreatic cancer, one of the most deadly and "incurable" cancers in the realm of conventional oncology, and scheduled for surgery. However, he had a heart attack as a side effect of a presurgical procedure he was undergoing, which caused his cancer surgery to get delayed. Within four weeks of his heart attack, while he was recovering from the cardiac event, the symptoms and laboratory findings of his pancreatic cancer began to resolve. Four months after the initial diagnosis, a CT scan revealed that his tumor had disappeared completely—without surgery, chemotherapy, or any other cancer treatment.

Four other case studies in the medical literature report "spontaneous" remissions from inoperable pancreatic cancers.[6,7] So what happened? Nowhere in these case studies do doctors explain why these cancers just disappeared.

Did these cancer patients find the root causes of their illness and clear those blockages so the body's natural cancer-fighting mechanisms could do their job? Did they finally find and fulfill their calling like Andy Mackie did? Did they fall in love and bathe their bodies with the naturally healing "molecules of emotion" that Candace Pert writes about? Did they pray for help from a higher power, start meditating, and experience a spiritual awakening that reorganized their entire physical, mental, emotional, spiritual, and energetic bodies? Did they join a healing circle and cure their loneliness? Did they start using food as medicine? Did they start dosing themselves with beauty baths in nature? Did they visit an energy healer and get their "chakras" rebalanced? Did they finally paint the masterpiece they'd been meaning to paint their whole life? What tools in the medicine toolbox did they put on their Prescriptions? Why didn't the doctors who wrote up these case studies ask them?

Maybe these patients who were cured from "incurable" pancreatic cancers were like Susannah, who was diagnosed with stage 4 endometrial cancer. Doctors gave her no hope. Although they surgically removed her uterus, fallopian tubes, and ovaries, as well as treating her with chemotherapy and radiation, her cancer recurred—twice. She tried many CAM treatments and was treated in clinics in Germany and Mexico. Finally, she sought out trauma treatment with AIT. She was treated for her cancer-prone "type C Personality," being dominated in her marriage, spiritual blockage, and a poorly functioning immune system. She went into remission after treatment and has been in remission for several years now.

Maybe those patients were like Genevieve, who was diagnosed with "incurable" Hashimoto's thyroiditis and told she would require thyroid replacement for the rest of her life. Not willing to accept the certainty of her doctor's prognosis, Genevieve sought out a trauma therapist who, over the course of a few days, helped her clear the traumas related to the root causes of her illness. Her thyroid normalized almost overnight, and she's now off all hormone replacement.

Or maybe they were like my client, whom I'll call Alicia. Alicia was a young nurse practitioner who had end-stage right-sided congestive heart failure as the result of pulmonary arterial hypertension secondary to the autoimmune disease scleroderma. Because of the underlying scleroderma, she was told she was not a candidate for heart/lung transplant because the scleroderma was likely to destroy the transplants too. She was given three to five years to live and encouraged to get her affairs in order. When I first met her, she was oxygen-dependent, weak, and barely able to walk because her exercise tolerance was so low.

Then Alicia heard about the Six Steps to Healing Yourself and decided to throw herself all the way into her healing journey, which included conventional pharmaceuticals, functional medicine, diet and nutrition changes, psychedelic plant medicine journeys, increasing how much sleep she was getting, psychotherapy, and many other CAM modalities. She also became a Whole Health Medicine Institute practitioner and now runs an integrative medicine practice that includes hypnotherapy, reiki, acupuncture, homeopathy, biofeedback, nutritional counseling, meditation practices, and sound/music therapy. A year after she completed her Whole Health Medicine Institute training, she burst into the retreat center where I was leading the next year's class and brandished her echocardiogram like a victory flag. Her heart and lung function was normal!

We even went hiking together up a mountain so she could prove her exercise tolerance. She took her last drug two years ago, and she's feeling great. Although she's still being monitored, her cardiopulmonary condition has not recurred.

Living a Whole Health Life

I sometimes wonder what my father would have thought about all of these patients who had radical remissions. In spite of his skepticism and dogged attachment to his worldview, it's hard to argue with reality. Before the first edition of this book was published, I hugged Mom and mused about what my very conventional physician, hard-nosed scientist, "woo" allergic father would think about this book if he had read it. The whole time I researched it, his voice was the voice in the back of my head, questioning me, prodding me, pushing me to go deeper, serving as the ultimate skeptic whose mind I was seeking to open and whose point of view I was hoping to expand.

I finally got up the nerve to ask my mother what she thought. If Dad were still alive, what would he think about what I was learning and writing about?

Mom was quiet and reflective. A tear formed in the corner of one eye. Then she smiled a crooked, sweet smile and told me that at first, he would have thought I'd gone off the deep end. But at some point, I would have appealed to the scientist in him. In the end, she suspected that even Dad would have looked at the evidence, compelled to open his mind *just enough* to consider that maybe there was at least a grain of truth here.

When she said that, I started to cry.

"What I do know for sure," Mom said, "is that, if your father were here right now, he'd be incredibly proud."

In that moment, I missed my father so much that I could feel my heart, right under my left breast, hollow and raw and sore and at the same time, full and overflowing. I confessed to Mom that I wrote this whole book to my father. His were the eyes on the other side of the page as I wrote. Perhaps if I could write a book that even doctors like my father could read without instantly shooing it away, maybe I could make a real difference in how health care is received and delivered. Maybe I could serve out my calling to redefine health and help people heal in a whole new way. Maybe I could attract a tribe of doctors and patients and other health-care providers who know our system is broken and long to reclaim the heart of medicine. Maybe I could teach people how to take responsibility for their health and bring the sacred back to the practice of medicine. Maybe—just maybe—I could help heal my beloved profession.

As the fictional physician character in Dr. Abraham Verghese's *Cutting for Stone* states, "We come unbidden into this life, and if we are lucky, we find a purpose beyond starvation, misery, and early death which, lest we forget, is the common lot. I grew up and I found my purpose, and it was to become a physician. My intent wasn't to save the world as much as to heal myself. Few doctors will admit this, certainly not young ones, but subconsciously, in entering the profession, we must believe that ministering to others will heal our woundedness. And it can. But it can also deepen the wound."

I was one of those doctors for whom the wound was deepened, and it made my body sick. But now, having learned how to heal myself, I long to help others do the same. The biggest lesson I've learned is that you can spend your life running scared and clinging to the illusion of control, grasping for what you think is certain until your life—and your health—suddenly crumble around you. Or you can recognize that the only thing certain in life is uncertainty. Whether you fear uncertainty and let it trigger stress responses or embrace uncertainty and let it elicit relaxation responses is your choice. Personally, I've come to recognize the beauty in uncertainty. While one face of uncertainty is the vast, scary unknown, the flip side of uncertainty is infinite possibility. When you don't know what the future holds, anything can happen.

These days, when I wake up in the morning, I'm fully aware that I have no idea what lies before me. Sure, I have a calendar filled with events, but events change, new opportunities arise, and my schedule has become fluid. What I thought I would be doing this year is different than what I anticipated a year ago. In fact, it's better than anything I could have even dreamed. Which is good news. It means that next year could hold even more gems I don't yet know to include in my fantasies. The world is my oyster. The sky's the limit. Look out, world.

The same is true for you. While you may feel fearful because you don't know what the future holds (especially if you're sick), anything could happen to you tomorrow. You could go to sleep tonight sick and wake up cured. Your symptoms could disappear forever. Your mood could lift. The love of your life could be standing behind you in Starbucks. The deal could come through. The house of your dreams could land in your lap. You could finally get pregnant. You could win the lottery. Your long-lost mother could show up. Violence around the world could come to a screeching halt. The seas could part in front of your very eyes.

If you are well and you've gone through these steps as a way to prevent disease in your life, high five to you! I applaud you for your courage and firmly believe you've just extended your life. And if you've done this because you're sick, high-fives to you too!

This is your precious life. Savor it. Grab the ring on the carousel. Ride the roller coaster. Do cartwheels. Open your heart. Never leave love unexpressed. Forgive generously. Love all your parts. Give openly. Heal your trauma. Follow your dream. Speak your truth. Sing and dance. Comfort your fear. Take leaps of faith. Make beautiful things. Serve those less fortunate. Honor what you desire. Prioritize pleasure. Let your freak flag fly. Surround yourself with those who love and accept you just the way you are. Live daringly. Be unapologetically you. It's preventive medicine. And it just might save your life.

APPENDIX A

8 Tips for How to Be in Your Body

1. Focus on a body part. Notice your right fingertip or your left knee or any other body part. How does it feel? Does it hurt? Is it cool or warm? Do you feel a breeze? Notice how it feels when you stroke it with a feather or brush it against the carpet. Pay attention to all your senses.

2. Name your sensation. Although words come from the mind, they can help connect the mind and the body by giving a name to what you feel. Be specific with the words you choose—does your body part feel stiff, loose, light, heavy, tingly, warm, cold, sensitive, numb, strong, weak, painful? Try to avoid describing your sensation in general terms such as "good" or "bad." Perhaps you feel clenched or spacious or prickly or heavy. Be as multisensory as you can.

3. Practice movement. Dancing, yoga, hiking, cycling, skiing, and other such physical activity can make you more aware of your body—what feels yummy and what hurts! Even pain can be a teacher about body awareness, so don't be afraid to lean into what you feel.

4. Use the floor. If you're having trouble feeling your body in space, try rolling around on the floor. It gives your body something to be in relationship with.

5. Optimize clothing. Wearing loose-fitting clothes that brush against your skin when you move can help you notice your body. If you wear tight-fitting clothes, you

may notice your body less than if you wear free-flowing pants or skirts and shirts with loose sleeves.

6. Get sexual. Nothing like a good romp in the hay to help you notice your body!

7. When trying to make a decision, notice how your body is responding. That guy who asked you out? How does your body feel—light or heavy? New job offer? Does your body feel open or closed? Your body is your compass. Pay attention.

8. Breathe. When you pay attention to your breathing, it helps center you in your body.

APPENDIX B

10 Factors That Support Radical Remission*

1. Radically changing your diet. Many radical remission survivors adopted a diet consisting primarily of whole vegetables, fruits, grains, and beans, while eliminating meat, sugar, dairy, and refined grains.

2. Taking control of your health. Rather than passively giving their power away to doctors or other practitioners, these patients took responsibility for their healing journey, researching their options, challenging authority, and making it a full-time job to be the empowered master of their experience, rather than a passive, compliant victim who blindly obeys doctor's orders without questioning their recommendations.

3. Following your intuition. Patients with radical remissions tuned into their intuition and trusted this inner guidance to help them make treatment decisions and lifestyle choices.

4. Using herbs and supplements. Many were taking immune-boosting and other supplements that they believed had the power to help cure their cancer; however, no single supplement or herb stood out.

5. Releasing suppressed emotions. Healing often called for these patients to openly feel, express, move through, and clear emotions they had suppressed, such as rage, grief, resentment, or fear.

6. Increasing positive emotions. These patients were proactive about gratitude practices, seeking out fun or humorous experiences, adding more love to their lives, and dosing up on pleasure, play, and laughter.

7. Embracing social support. Those who experienced radical remissions stopped obsessively caregiving others and opened themselves to receiving love, allowing others to rally to support them through their crisis, rather than suffering in silence or refusing help.

8. Deepening your spiritual connection. Many used their cancer as a wake-up call and prioritized regular spiritual practices and experiences, which fostered spiritual awakenings, mystical experiences, and other spiritual phenomena that heightened their attunement to invisible forces of love in the spiritual realm.

9. Having strong reasons for living. Those who felt a strong mission to serve, had a child they wanted to raise, fell in love with a new partner, or otherwise felt that there was unfinished business in this life experienced a strong will to live that fueled healing.

10. Regular exercise. Moving the body became a priority.

* Excerpted from *Radical Remission*, by Kelly Turner, Ph.D. The 10th factor emerged after publication of the book, as Dr. Turner has kept up her research.

CONTINUE YOUR SELF-HEALING JOURNEY

- To download a free Self-Healing Kit designed by Lissa Rankin to support your healing journey, visit MindOverMedicineBook.com

- If you're a practitioner interested in being certified to facilitate the Six Steps to Healing Yourself, visit WholeHealthMedicineInstitute.com

- For other free self-healing resources, visit LissaRankin.com/free-healing

- To keep updated on self-healing tools, subscribe to Lissa Rankin's blog at LissaRankin.com or follow her on Facebook, Twitter, and Instagram

- To deepen your connection to your Inner Pilot Light as a way of strengthening your Whole Health Cairn work, sign up for the free Daily Flame at InnerPilotLight.com

- To commune online with others who are practicing the Six Steps to Healing Yourself, visit HealingSoulTribe.com

- To keep informed about the Heal At Last project or find a healing circle near you, visit HealAtLast.org

- To get help treating your traumas with Internal Family Systems (IFS) or find an IFS therapist, visit IFS-institute.com

- To get help treating your traumas with Advanced Integrative Therapy (AIT) or find an AIT therapist, visit AIT.institute
- For inspiration from the Radical Remission Project of Kelly Turner, Ph.D., visit RadicalRemission.com

ENDNOTES

Introduction

1. Dan Buettner, "The Island where People Forget to Die," *The New York Times Magazine* online, October 24, 2012, https://www.nytimes.com/2012/10/28/magazine/the-island-where-people-forget-to-die.html.

2. Anne Harrington, *The Cure Within: A History of Mind-Body Medicine* (New York: W. W. Norton & Company, 2008), 250–51.

3. Patrick Cooke, "They Cried until They Could Not See," *New York Times Magazine,* June 23, 1991.

4. Simon G. Talbot and Wendy Dean, "Physicians aren't 'burning out.' They're suffering from moral injury," First Opinion, *STAT,* July 26, 2018, https://www.statnews.com/2018/07/26/physicians-not-burning-out-they-are-suffering-moral-injury/.

Chapter 1

1. Bruno Klopfer, "Psychological Variables in Human Cancer," *Journal of Projective Techniques* 21, no. 4 (December 1957): 331–40.

2. Stewart Wolf, "The Effects of Suggestion and Conditioning on the Action of Chemical Agents in Human Subjects: The Pharmacology of Placebos," *The Journal of Clinical Investigation* 29, no. 1 (January 1950): 100–109.

3. J. Bruce Moseley et al., "A Controlled Trial of Arthroscopic Surgery for Osteoarthritis of the Knee," *New England Journal of Medicine* 347 (July 11, 2002): 81–88.

4. Margaret Talbot, "The Placebo Prescription," *New York Times Magazine,* January 9, 2000.

5. Henry K. Beecher, "The Powerful Placebo," *Journal of the American Medical Association* 159, no. 17 (December 24, 1955): 1602–6.

6. Michael E. Wechsler et al., "Active Albuterol or Placebo, Sham Acupuncture, or No Intervention in Asthma," *New England Journal of Medicine* 365 (July 14, 2011): 119–26.

7. Femke M. de Groot et al., "Headache: The Placebo Effects in the Control Groups in Randomized Clinical Trials; An Analysis of Systematic Reviews," *Journal of Manipulative and Physiological Therapeutics* 34, no. 5 (June 2011): 297–305.

8. Talbot, "The Placebo Prescription."

9. H. J. Binder et al., "Cimetidine in the Treatment of Duodenal Ulcer: A Multicenter Double Blind Study," *Gastroenterology* 74 (February 1978): 380–88.

10. Shirley S. Wang, "Why Placebos Work Wonders," *Wall Street Journal,* January 10, 2012, http://online.wsj.com/article/SB1000142405297020472020457712887388864 71982.html.

11. F. J. Evans, "Expectancy, Therapeutic Instructions, and the Placebo Response," in *Placebo: Theory, Research and Mechanisms,* ed. Leonard White, Bernard Tursky, and Gary E. Schwartz (New York: Guilford Press, 1985); J. D. Levine et al., "Analgesic Responses to Morphine and Placebo in Individuals with Postoperative Pain," *Pain* 10, no. 3 (June 1981): 379–89.

12. Irving Kirsch, *The Emperor's New Drugs: Exploding the Antidepressant Myth* (New York: Basic Books, 2010); Irving Kirsch and Guy Sapirstein, "Listening to Prozac but Hearing Placebo: A Meta-Analysis of Antidepressant Medication," *Prevention & Treatment* 1, no. 2 (June 1998); Shankar Vedantam, "Against Depression, a Sugar Pill Is Hard to Beat: Placebos Improve Mood, Change Brain Chemistry in Majority of Trials of Antidepressants," *Washington Post,* May 7, 2002; Arif Khan et al., "Suicide Rates in Clinical Trials of SSRIs, Other Antidepressants, and Placebo: Analysis of FDA Reports," *The American Journal of Psychiatry* 160, no. 4 (April 1, 2003): 790–92.

13. Judith A. Turner et al., "The Importance of Placebo Effects in Pain Treatment and Research," *Journal of the American Medical Association* 271, no. 20 (May 25, 1994): 1609–14; Leonard A. Cobb et al., "An Evaluation of Internal-Mammary-Artery Ligation by a Double-Blind Technic," *New England Journal of Medicine,* 260, no. 22 (May 28, 1959): 1115–18.

14. Andrew L. Geers et al., "Dispositional Optimism Predicts Placebo Analgesia," *The Journal of Pain* 11, no. 11 (November 2010): 1165–71, https://doi.org/10.1016/j.jpain.2010.02.014.

15. Marta Peciña et al., "Personality Trait Predictors of Placebo Analgesia and Neurobiological Correlates," *Neuropsychopharmacology* 38 (November 16, 2012): 639–46, https://doi.org/10.1038/npp.2012.227.

16. Elise A. Olsen et al., "A Multicenter, Randomized, Placebo-Controlled, Double-Blind Clinical Trial of a Novel Formulation of 5% Minoxidil Topical Foam Versus Placebo in the Treatment of Androgenetic Alopecia in Men," *Journal of the American Academy of Dermatology* 57, no. 5 (November 2007): 767–74; Richard A. Preston et al., "Placebo-Associated Blood Pressure Response and Adverse Effects in the Treatment of Hypertension: Observations from a Department of Veterans Affairs Cooperative Study," *Archives of Internal Medicine* 160, no. 10 (May 22, 2000): 1449–54; H. V. Allington, "Review of the Psychotherapy of Warts," *AMA Archives of Dermatology and Syphilology* 66, no. 3 (1952): 316–26; H. Vollmer, "Treatment of Warts by Suggestion," *Psychosomatic Medicine* 8 (March 1946): 138–42; Montague Ullman and Stephanie Dudek, "On the Psyche and Warts: Hypnotic Suggestion and Warts," *Psychosomatic Medicine* 22, no. 1 (January 1, 1960): 437–88; Anton J. M. De Craen et al., "Placebo Effect in the Treatment of Duodenal Ulcer," *British Journal of Clinical Pharmacology* 48, no. 6 (December 1999): 853–60; F. K. Abbot, M. Mack, and S. Wolf, "The Action of Banthine on

the Stomach and Duodenum of Man with Observations on the Effects of Placebos," *Gastroenterology* 20, no. 2 (February 1952): 249–61; Talbot, "The Placebo Prescription"; Paul L. Canner, Sandra A. Forman, and Gerard J. Prud'homme, "Influence of Adherence to Treatment and Response of Cholesterol on Mortality in the Coronary Drug Project," *New England Journal of Medicine* 303 (October 30, 1980): 1038–41; Ibrahim Hashish et al., "Reduction of Postoperative Pain and Swelling by Ultrasound Treatment: A Placebo Effect," *Pain* 33, no. 3 (June 1988): 303–11; Raúl de la Fuente-Fernández et al., "Expectation and Dopamine Release: Mechanism of the Placebo Effect in Parkinson's Disease," *Science* 293, no. 5532 (August 10, 2001): 1164–66; C. Kirschbaum et al., "Conditioning of Drug-Induced Immunomodulation in Human Volunteers: A European Collaborative Study," *British Journal of Clinical Psychology* 31, no. 4 (November 1992): 459–72; Predrag Petrovic et al., "Placebo and Opioid Analgesia: Imaging a Shared Neuronal Network," *Science* 295, no. 5560 (March 1, 2002): 1737–40; Matthew D. Lieberman et al., "The Neural Correlates of Placebo Effects: A Disruption Account," *Neuroimage* 22, no. 1 (May 2004): 447–55; Tor D. Wager et al., "Placebo-Induced Changes in fMRI in the Anticipation and Experience of Pain," *Science* 303, no. 5661 (February 20, 2004): 1162–67.

17. Irving Kirsch, "Response Expectancy as a Determinant of Experience and Behavior," *American Psychologist* 40, no. 11 (November 1985): 1189–1202.

18. I. Wickramasekera, "A Conditioned Response Model of the Placebo Effect: Predictions from the Model," *Biofeedback and Self-Regulation* 5, no. 1 (March 1980): 5–18; Nicholas J. Voudouris, Connie L. Peck, and Grahame Coleman, "Conditioned Response Models of Placebo Phenomena: Further Support," *Pain* 38, no. 1 (July 1989): 109–16.

19. D. G. Finniss et al., "Biological, Clinical, and Ethical Advances of Placebo Effects," *The Lancet* 375, no. 9715 (February 20, 2010): 686–95, https://doi.org/10.1016/S0140-6736(09)61706-2.

20. Asbjørn Hróbjartsson and Peter C. Gøtzsche, "Is the Placebo Powerless? An Analysis of Clinical Trials Comparing Placebo with No Treatment," *New England Journal of Medicine* 344, no. 21 (May 24, 2001): 1594–1602.

21. Daniel E. Moerman and Wayne B. Jonas, "Deconstructing the Placebo Effect and Finding the Meaning Response," *Annals of Internal Medicine* 136, no. 6 (March 19, 2002): 471–76.

22. Fabrizio Benedetti, *Placebo Effects: Understanding the Mechanisms in Health and Disease* (New York: Oxford University Press, 2009): 29.

23. Ted J. Kaptchuk and Franklin G. Miller, "Placebo Effects in Medicine," Perspective, *New England Journal of Medicine* 373 (July 2, 2015): 8–9, https://doi.org/10.1056/NEJMp1504023.

24. Harvard Health Publishing, "The Power of the Placebo Effect," Harvard Men's Health Watch, Harvard University, updated August 9, 2019, https://www.health.harvard.edu/mental-health/the-power-of-the-placebo-effect.

25. Jon D. Levine, Newton C. Gordon, and Howard L. Fields, "The Mechanism of Placebo Analgesia," *Lancet* 312, no. 8091 (September 23, 1978): 654–57.

26. R. Ader and N. Cohen, "Behaviorally Conditioned Immunosuppression," *Psychosomatic Medicine* 37, no. 4 (July/August 1975): 333–40.

27. Evans, *Placebo: Mind over Matter in Modern Medicine,* 44–69.

28. Benedetti et al., "Loss of Expectation-Related Mechanisms in Alzheimer's Disease Makes Analgesic Therapies Less Effective."

29. David J. Scott et al., "Individual Differences in Reward Responding Explain Placebo-Induced Expectations and Effects," *Neuron* 55, no. 2 (July 19, 2007): 325–36.

30. http://cancer.org/treatment/treatments-and-side-effects/clinical-trials/placebo-effect.html.

31. Ted J. Kaptchuk and Franklin G. Miller, "Placebo Effects in Medicine," Perspective, *New England Journal of Medicine* 373 (July 2, 2015): 8–9, https://doi.org/10.1056/NEJMp1504023.

32. Caryle Hirshberg and Brendan O'Regan, *Spontaneous Remission: An Annotated Bibliography* (Petaluma, CA: Institute of Noetic Sciences, 1993), http://noetic.org/library/publication-books/spontaneous-remission-annotated-bibliography/.

33. Ibid.

34. https://exponential.singularityu.org/medicine/faculty2017/jeffrey-d-rediger/.

Chapter 2

1. D. P. Phillips, T. E. Ruth, and L. M. Wagner, "Psychology and Survival," *Lancet* 342, no. 8880 (November 6, 1993): 1142–45.

2. S. M. Woods, J. Natterson, and J. Silverman, "Medical Students' Disease: Hypochondriasis in Medical Education," *Journal of Medical Education* 41, no. 8 (August 1966): 785–90.

3. Bernie S. Siegel, *Love, Medicine & Miracles* (New York: Harper & Row, 1986), 133.

4. Pierre Kissel and Dominique Barrucand, *Placebos et Effet Placebo en Médecine* (Paris: Masson, 1964).

5. Avraham Schweiger and Allen Parducci, "Nocebo: The Psychologic Induction of Pain," *Pavlovian Journal of Biological Science* 16, no. 3 (July–September 1981): 140–43.

6. Brian Reid, "The Nocebo Effect: The Placebo Effect's Evil Twin," *The Washington Post,* April 30, 2002.

7. Ibid.

8. Anthony Robbins, *Unlimited Power: The New Science of Personal Achievement* (New York: Free Press, 1986).

9. Bennett G. Braun, ed., *The Treatment of Multiple Personality Disorder* (Arlington, VA: American Psychiatric Press, 1986).

10. Richard L. Kradin, *The Placebo Response and the Power of Unconscious Healing* (New York: Routledge, 2008), 151.

11. Martina Amanzio et al., "A Systematic Review of Adverse Events in Placebo Groups of Anti-migraine Clinical Trials," *Pain* 146, no. 3 (December 5, 2009): 261–69.

12. Walter B. Cannon, "Voodoo Death," *American Anthropologist* 44, no. 2 (April–June, 1942): 169–81.

13. John Cloud, "The Flip Side of Placebos: The Nocebo Effect," *Time,* October 13, 2009.

14. Sanford I. Cohen, "Voodoo Death, the Stress Response, and AIDS," *Advanced Biochemical Psychopharmacology* 44 (1998): 95–109.

15. D. N. Ruble, "Premenstrual Symptoms: A Reinterpretation," *Science* 197, no. 4300 (July 15, 1977): 291–292.

16. Michael J. Colligan and Lawrence R. Murphy, "Mass Psychogenic Illness in Organizations: An Overview," *Journal of Occupational Psychology* 52, no. 2 (June 1979): 77–90.

17. Fabrizio Benedetti et al., "The Biochemical and Neuroendocrine Bases of the Hyperalgesic Nocebo Effect," *Journal of Neuroscience* 26, no. 46 (November 15, 2006): 12014–22.

18. Bruce Lipton, *The Biology of Belief: Unleashing the Power of Consciousness, Matter and Miracles* (Carlsbad, CA: Hay House, 2008).

19. Robert A. Waterland and Randy L. Jirtle, "Transposable Elements: Targets for Early Nutritional Effects on Epigenetic Gene Regulation," *Molecular and Cellular Biology* 23, no. 15 (August 2003): 5293–5300; Eva Jablonka and Marion J. Lamb, *Epigenetic Inheritance and Evolution: The Lamarckian Dimension* (Oxford: Oxford University Press, 1995).

20. Walter C. Willett, "Balancing Life-Style and Genomics Research for Disease Prevention," *Science* 296, no. 5568 (April 26, 2002): 695–98.

21. Peter D. Gluckman and Mark A. Hanson, "Living with the Past: Evolution, Development, and Patterns of Disease," *Science* 305, no. 5691 (September 17, 2004): 1733–36.

22. Peter W. Nathanielsz, *Life in the Womb: The Origin of Health and Disease* (New York: Promethean Press, 1999).

23. James W. Prescott, Scientific Director, *Rock A Bye Baby* (New York: Time-Life Films, 1970).

24. Patrick Bateson et al., "Developmental Plasticity and Human Health," *Nature* 430, no. 6998 (July 22, 2004): 419–21.

Chapter 3

1. "One Scholar's Take on the Power of the Placebo," *Science Friday,* NPR, January 6, 2012, http://m.npr.org/news/Health/144794035.

2. Michael Specter, "The Power of Nothing," *New Yorker,* December 12, 2011.

3. Michael E. Wechsler et al., "Active Albuterol or Placebo, Sham Acupuncture, or No Intervention in Asthma," *New England Journal of Medicine* 365 (July 14, 2011): 119–26.

4. Lawrence D. Egbert et al., "Reduction of Postoperative Pain by Encouragement and Instruction of Patients: A Study of Doctor-Patient Rapport," *New England Journal of Medicine* 270 (April 16, 1964): 825–27.

5. Ibid.

6. K. B. Thomas, "General Practice Consultations: Is There Any Point in Being Positive?" *British Medical Journal* 294, no. 6581 (May 9, 1987): 1200–1202.

7. Fabrizio Benedetti et al., "When Words Are Painful: Unraveling the Mechanisms of the Nocebo Effect," *Neuroscience* 147, no. 2 (June 29, 2007): 260–71.

8. Richard H. Gracely et al., "Clinicians' Expectations Influence Placebo Analgesia," *Lancet* 325, no. 8419 (January 5, 1985): 43.

9. Janice L. Krupnick et al., "The Role of the Therapeutic Alliance in Psychotherapy and Pharmacotherapy Outcome: Findings in the National Institute of Mental Health Treatment of Depression Collaborative Research Program," *Journal of Consulting and Clinical Psychology* 64, no. 3 (June 1996): 532–39.

10. Ted J. Kaptchuk et al., "Components of Placebo Effect: Randomised Controlled Trial in Patients with Irritable Bowel Syndrome," *British Medical Journal* 336, no. 7651 (May 1, 2008): 999–1003.

11. A. H. Sinclair-Gieben and D. Chalmers, "Evaluation of Treatment of Warts by Hypnosis," *Lancet* 274, no. 7101 (October 3, 1959): 480–82; Owen S. Surman, Sheldon K. Gottlieb, and Thomas P. Hackett, "Hypnotic Treatment of a Child with Warts," *American Journal of Clinical Hypnosis* 15, no. 1 (July 1972): 12–14.

12. Curtis E. Margo, "The Placebo Effect," *Survey of Ophthalmology* 44, no. 1 (July/August 1999): 33–34; Nicholas J. Voudouris, Connie L. Peck, and Grahame Coleman, "Conditioned Response Models of Placebo Phenomena: Further Support," *Pain* 38, no. 1 (July 1989): 109–16; Steve Stewart-Williams and John Podd, "The Placebo Effect: Dissolving the Expectancy Versus Conditioning Debate," *Psychology Bulletin* 130, no. 2 (March 2004): 324–40.

13. Patricia Leigh Brown, "A Doctor for Disease, a Shaman for the Soul," *The New York Times*, September 19, 2009, https://www.nytimes.com/2009/09/20/us/20shaman.html.

14. Desonta Holder, "Health: Beware Negative Self-Fulfilling Prophecy," *Seattle Times*, January 2, 2008, https://www.seattletimes.com/seattle-news/health/health-beware-negative-self-fulfilling-prophecy.

15. David Spiegel and Anne Harrington, "What Is the Placebo Worth?" *British Medical Journal* 336, no. 7651 (May 3, 2008): 967–68.

Chapter 4

1. Richard A. Dienstbier, "Arousal and Physiological Toughness: Implications for Mental and Physical Health," *Psychological Review* 96, no. 1 (January 1989): 84–100; Marianne Frankenhaeuser, "The Psychophysiology of Workload,

Stress, and Health: Comparison Between the Sexes," *Annals of Behavioral Medicine* 13, no. 4 (1991): 197–204; Shelley E. Taylor, *Health Psychology* (New York: McGraw-Hill, 1999), 168–201.

2. Andrew H. Kemp and Daniel S. Quintana, "The Relationship between Mental and Physical Health: Insights from the Study of Heart Rate Variability," *International Journal of Psychophysiology* 89, no. 3 (September 2013): 288–96.

Chapter 5

1. Malcolm Gladwell, *Outliers: The Story of Success* (New York: Little, Brown & Company, 2008), 7.

2. J. S. House, K. R. Landis, and D. Umberson, "Social Relationships and Health," *Science* 241, no. 4865 (July 29, 1988): 540–45.

3. Ron Grossman and Charles Leroux, "A New 'Roseto Effect': 'People Are Nourished by Other People,'" *Chicago Tribune*, October 11, 1996, http://articles.chicagotribune .com/1996-10-11/news/9610110254_1_satellite-dishes-outsiders-town/2.

4. Lisa F. Berkman and S. Leonard Syme, "Social Networks, Host Resistance, and Mortality: A Nine-Year Follow-Up Study of Alameda County Residents," *American Journal of Epidemiology* 109, no. 2 (February 1, 1979): 186–204.

5. Peggy Reynolds and George A. Kaplan, "Social Connections and Risk for Cancer: Prospective Evidence from the Alameda County Study," *Behavioral Medicine* 16, no. 3 (Fall 1990): 101–10.

6. Thomas A. Glass et al., "Population Based Study of Social and Productive Activities as Predictors of Survival among Elderly Americans," *British Medical Journal* 319 (August 21, 1999): 478.

7. L. C. Giles et al., "Effect of Social Networks on 10 Year Survival in Very Old Australians: The Australian Longitudinal Study of Aging," *Journal of Epidemiological Community Health* 59, no. 7 (July 2005): 574–79; J. S. House, C. Robbins, and H. L. Metzner, "The Association of Social Relationships and Activities with Mortality: Prospective Evidence from the Tecumseh Community Health Study," *American Journal of Epidemiology* 116, no. 1 (July 1982): 123–40.

8. Candyce H. Kroenke et al., "Social Networks, Social Support, and Survival after Breast Cancer Diagnosis," *Journal of Clinical Oncology* 24, no. 7 (March 1, 2006): 1105–11.

9. Annika Rosengren, Lars Wilhelmsen, and Kristina Orth-Gomér, "Coronary Disease in Relation to Social Support and Social Class in Swedish Men: A 15 Year Follow-Up in the Study of Men Born in 1933," *European Heart Journal* 25, no. 1 (January 2004): 56–63.

10. Jo Marchant, "Heal Thyself: Trust People," *NewScientist,* August 24, 2011, https:// www.newscientist.com/article/mg21128271.800-heal-thyself-trust-people.html.

11. W. J. Strawbridge et al., "Frequent Attendance at Religious Services and Mortality over 28 Years," *American Journal of Public Health* 87, no. 6 (June 1997): 957–61.

12. D. Oman and D. Reed, "Religion and Mortality among the Community-Dwelling Elderly," *American Journal of Public Health* 88, no. 10 (October 1998): 1469–75.

13. T. E. Oxman, D. H. Freeman, and E. D. Manheimer, "Lack of Social Participation or Religious Strength and Comfort as Risk Factors for Death after Cardiac Surgery in the Elderly," *Psychosomatic Medicine* 57, no. 1 (January/February 1995): 5–15.

14. Harold G. Koenig et al., "Modeling the Cross-Sectional Relationships Between Religion, Physical Health, Social Support, and Depressive Symptoms," *American Journal of Geriatric Psychology* 5, no. 2 (Spring 1997): 131–44.

15. Christopher G. Ellison and Jeffrey S. Levin, "The Religion-Health Connection: Evidence, Theory, and Future Directions," *Health Education and Behavior* 25, no. 6 (December 1998): 700–720.

16. Robert A. Hummer et al., "Religious Involvement and U.S. Adult Mortality," *Demography* 36, no. 2 (May 1999): 273–85; Michael E. McCullough et al., "Religious Involvement and Mortality: A Meta-Analytic Review," *Health Psychology* 19, no. 3 (May 2000): 211–22.

17. Patrick R. Steffen et al., "Religious Coping, Ethnicity, and Ambulatory Blood Pressure," *Psychosomatic Medicine* 63, no. 4 (July–August 2001): 523–30; John Gartner, Dave B. Larson, and George D. Allen, "Religious Commitment and Mental Health: A Review of the Empirical Literature," *Journal of Psychology and Theology* 19, no. 1 (Spring 1991): 6–25; Harold G. Koenig and David B. Larson, "Religion and Mental Health: Evidence for an Association," *International Review of Psychiatry* 13, no. 2 (2001): 67–78; Sandra E. Sephton et al., "Spiritual Expression and Immune Status in Women with Metastatic Breast Cancer: An Exploratory Study," *Breast Journal* 7, no. 5 (September/October 2001): 345–53; Teresa E. Woods et al., "Religiosity Is Associated with Affective and Immune Status in Symptomatic HIV-Infected Gay Men," *Journal of Psychosomatic Research* 46, no. 2 (February 1999): 165–76.

18. Joseph L. Lyon, Kent Gardner, and Richard E. Gress, "Cancer Incidence in Mormons and Non-Mormons in Utah (United States) 1971–1985," *Cancer Causes & Control* 5, no. 2 (March 1994): 149–56.

19. William J. Strawbridge, Richard D. Cohen, and Sarah J. Shema, "Comparative Strength of Association between Religious Attendance and Survival," *International Journal of Psychiatry in Medicine* 30, no. 4 (2000): 299–308; Doug Oman et al., "Religious Attendance and Cause of Death Over 31 Years," *International Journal of Psychiatry in Medicine* 32, no. 1 (2002): 69–89.

20. Daniel N. McIntosh, Roxane Cohen Silver, and Camille B. Wortman, "Religion's Role in Adjustment to a Negative Life Event: Coping with the Loss of a Child," *Journal of Personality and Social Psychology* 65, no. 4 (October 1993): 812–21.

21. Michael E. McCullough and Everett L. Worthington, Jr., "Religion and the Forgiving Personality," *Journal of Personality* 67, no. 6 (December 1999): 1141–64.

22. Melvin Pollner, "Divine Relations, Social Relations, and Well-Being," *Journal of Health and Social Behavior* 30 no. 1 (March 1989): 92–104.

23. Kenneth I. Pargament, "The Psychology of Religion and Spirituality?: Yes and No," *International Journal for the Psychology of Religion* 9, no. 1 (1999): 3–16.

24. Harold G. Koenig, Kenneth I. Pargament, and Julie Nielsen, "Religious Coping and Health Status in Medically Ill Hospitalized Older Adults," *Journal of Nervous and Mental Disease* 186, no. 9 (September 1998): 513–21.

25. Pamela Kotler and Deborah Lee Wingard, "The Effect of Occupational, Marital and Parental Roles on Mortality: The Alameda County Study," *American Journal of Public Health* 79, no. 5 (May 1989): 607–12.

26. Robert M. Kaplan and Richard G. Kronick, "Marital Status and Longevity in the United States Population," *Journal of Epidemiology and Community Health* 60, no. 9 (September 2006): 760–65.

27. Brigham Young University, "Happily Marrieds Have Lower Blood Pressure Than Social Singles," *ScienceDaily,* March 21, 2008, http://www.sciencedaily.com/releases/2008/03/080320192610.htm.

28. American Academy of Sleep Medicine, "More Marital Happiness = Less Sleep Complaints," *ScienceDaily,* June 11, 2008, http://www.sciencedaily.com/releases/2008/06/080609071336.htm.

29. Sheree J. Gibb, David M. Fergusson, and L. John Horwood, "Relationship Duration and Mental Health Outcomes: Findings from a 30-Year Longitudinal Study," *British Journal of Psychiatry* 198, no. 1 (2011): 24–30.

30. Dario Maestripieri et al., "Between- and Within-Sex Variation in Hormonal Responses to Psychological Stress in a Large Sample of College Students," *Stress* 13, no. 5 (September 2010): 413–24; "Relationships Are Good for Your Health: Being Married or in a Long-Term Relationship Improves Your Ability to Deal with Stress, a New Study Suggests," *Telegraph,* August 18, 2010, http://www.telegraph.co.uk/health/healthnews/7952466/Relationships-are-good-for-your-health.html.

31. BMJ–British Medical Journal, "Marriage Is Good for Physical and Mental Health, Study Finds," *ScienceDaily,* January 28, 2011, http://www.sciencedaily.com/releases/2011/01/110127205853.htm.

32. Ohio State University, "Marital Problems Lead to Poorer Outcomes for Breast Cancer Patients," *ScienceDaily,* December 10, 2008, http://www.sciencedaily.com/releases/2008/12/081208123304.htm.

33. Wiley-Blackwell, "Intimate Abuse Study Finds Clear Links with Poor Health and Calls for Holistic Primary Care Approach," *ScienceDaily,* July 6, 2009, http://www.sciencedaily.com/releases/2009/07/090706090438.htm.

34. James W. Pennebaker and Robin C. O'Heeron, "Confiding in Others and Illness Rate among Spouses of Suicide and Accidental-Death Victims," *Journal of Abnormal Psychology* 93, no. 4 (November 1984): 473–76.

35. George Davey Smith, Stephen Frankel, and John Yarnell, "Sex and Death: Are They Related? Findings from the Caerphilly Cohort Study," *British Medical Journal* 315, no. 7133 (December 20–27, 1997): 1641–44; Erdman B. Palmore, "Predictors of the Longevity Difference: A 25-Year Follow-Up," *Gerontologist* 22, no. 6 (December 1982): 513–18; G. Persson, "Five-Year Mortality in a 70-Year-Old Urban Population in Relation to Psychiatric Diagnosis, Personality, Sexuality and Early Parental Death," *Acta Psychiatrica Scandinavica* 64, no. 3 (September 1981): 244–53; S. Ebrahim et al., "Sexual Intercourse and Risk of Ischaemic Stroke and Coronary Heart Disease: The Caerphilly Study," *Journal of Epide-*

miology and Community Health 56, no. 2 (February 2002): 99–102; Monique G. Lê, Annie Bacheloti, and Catherine Hill, "Characteristics of Reproductive Life and Risk of Breast Cancer in a Case-Control Study of Young Nulliparous Women," *Journal of Clinical Epidemiology* 42, no. 12 (1989): 1227–33; Carl J. Charnetski and Francis X. Brennan, *Feeling Good Is Good for You: How Pleasure Can Boost Your Immune System and Lengthen Your Life* (Emmaus, PA: Rodale Books, 2001); Carol Rinkleib Ellison, *Women's Sexualities* (Oakland, CA: New Harbinger Publications, Inc., 2000); David Weeks and Jamie James, *Secrets of the Superyoung* (New York: Berkley Books, 1999); Winnifred B. Cutler, *Love Cycles: The Science of Intimacy* (New York: Villard Books, 1991); Helen Singer Kaplan, "Desire? Why and How It Changes," *Redbook,* October 1984, as cited in B. R. Komisaruk and B. Whipple, "The Suppression of Pain by Genital Stimulation in Females," *Annual Review of Sex Research* 6 (1995): 151–86; D. Shapiro, "Effect of Chronic Low Back Pain on Sexuality," *Medical Aspects of Human Sexuality* 17 (1983): 241–45, as cited in Komisaruk and Whipple, "The Suppression of Pain by Genital Stimulation in Females"; Beverly Whipple and Barry R. Komisaruk, "Elevation of Pain Threshold by Vaginal Stimulation in Women," *Pain* 21, no. 4 (April 1985): 357–67; Randolph W. Evans and James R. Couch, "Orgasm and Migraine," *Headache* 41, no. 5 (May 2001): 512–14; Joseph A. Catania and Charles B. White, "Sexuality in an Aged Sample: Cognitive Determinants of Masturbation," *Archives of Sexual Behavior* 11, no. 3 (June 1982): 237–45; David J. Weeks, "Sex for the Mature Adult: Health, Self-Esteem and Countering Ageist Stereotypes," *Sexual and Relationship Therapy* 17, no. 3 (2002): 231–40; Pamela Warner and John Bancroft, "Mood, Sexuality, Oral Contraceptives and the Menstrual Cycle," *Journal of Psychosomatic Research* 32, no. 4–5 (1988): 417–27; Edward O. Laumann et al., *The Social Organization of Sexuality: Sexual Practice in the United States* (Chicago: University of Chicago, 1994).

36. Leah Irish et al., "Long-term Physical Health Consequences of Childhood Sexual Abuse: A Meta-Analytic Review," *Journal of Pediatric Psychology* 35, no. 5 (June 2010): 450–61, https://www.doi.org/10.1093/jpepsy/jsp118.

37. Vello Sermat, "Some Situational and Personality Correlates of Loneliness," in *The Anatomy of Loneliness*, ed. Joseph Hartog, J. Ralph Audy, and Yehudi A. Cohen (New York: International Universities Press, 1980).

38. C. M. Rubenstein and P. Shaver, "Loneliness in Two Northeastern Cities," in Hartog et al. ed., *The Anatomy of Loneliness*.

39. Roelof Hortulanus, Anja Machielse, and Ludwien Meeuwesen, *Social Isolation in Modern Society* (New York: Routledge, 2004).

40. Robert D. Putnam, *Bowling Alone: The Collapse and Revival of American Community* (New York: Simon & Schuster, 2001).

41. John T. Cacioppo et al., "Loneliness and Health: Potential Mechanisms," *Psychosomatic Medicine* 64, no. 3 (May/June 2002): 407–17.

42. Andrew Steptoe et al., "Loneliness and Neuroendocrine, Cardiovascular, and Inflammatory Stress Responses in Middle-Aged Men and Women," *Psychoneuroendocrinology* 29, no. 5 (June 2004): 593–611.

43. Dara Sorkin, Karen S. Rook, and John L. Lu, "Loneliness, Lack of Emotional Support, Lack of Companionship, and the Likelihood of Having a Heart Condition in an Elderly Sample," *Annals of Behavioral Medicine* 24, no. 4 (Fall 2002): 290–98;

Cyndy M. Fox et al., "Loneliness, Emotional Repression, Marital Quality, and Major Life Events in Women Who Develop Breast Cancer," *Journal of Community Health* 19, no. 6 (December 1994): 467–82; Robert S. Wilson et al., "Loneliness and Risk of Alzheimer Disease," *Archives of General Psychiatry* 64, no. 2 (February 2007): 234–40; Ariel Stravynski and Richard Boyer, "Loneliness in Relation to Suicide Ideation and Parasuicide: A Population-Wide Study," *Suicide and Life-Threatening Behavior* 31, no. 1 (Spring 2001): 32–40.

44. J. Herlitz et al., "The Feeling of Loneliness prior to Coronary Artery Bypass Grafting Might Be a Predictor of Short- and Long-Term Postoperative Mortality," *European Journal of Vascular and Endovascular Surgery* 16, no. 2 (August 1998): 120–25.

45. Cacioppo et al., "Loneliness and Health: Potential Mechanisms."

46. John T. Cacioppo et al., "Lonely Traits and Concomitant Physiological Processes: The MacArthur Social Neuroscience Studies," *International Journal of Psychophysiology* 35, no. 2–3 (March 2000): 143–54.

47. Janice K. Kiecolt-Glaser et al., "Psychosocial Modifiers of Immunocompetence in Medical Students," *Psychosomatic Medicine* 46, no. 1 (January/February 1984): 7–14; Janice K. Kiecolt-Glaser et al., "Urinary Cortisol Levels, Cellular Immunocompetency, and Loneliness in Psychiatric Patients," *Psychosomatic Medicine* 46, no. 1 (January/February 1984): 15–23; Sarah D. Pressman et al., "Loneliness, Social Network Size, and Immune Response to Influenza Vaccination in College Freshmen," *Health Psychology* 24, no. 3 (May 2005): 297–306; Bert N. Uchino, John T. Cacioppo, and Janice K. Kiecolt-Glaser, "The Relationship between Support and Physiological Processes: A Review with Emphasis on Underlying Mechanisms and Implications for Health," *Psychological Bulletin* 119, no. 3 (May 1996): 488–531.

48. James J. Lynch, *The Broken Heart* (New York: Basic Books, 1977), 84.

49. Karen S. Rook, "The Negative Side of Social Interaction: Impact on Psychological Well-Being," *Journal of Personality and Social Psychology* 46, no. 5 (May 1984): 1097–1108.

50. Brené Brown, *The Gifts of Imperfection* (Center City, MN: Hazelden, 2010).

Chapter 6

1. K. Morioka, "Work Till You Drop," *New Labor Forum* 13, no. 1 (Spring 2004): 81–85.

2. Becky Barrow, "Stress 'Is Top Cause of Workplace Sickness' and Is So Widespread It's Dubbed the 'Black Death of the 21st Century,'" *MailOnline*, October 5, 2011, http://www.dailymail.co.uk/health/article-2045309/Stress-Top-cause-workplace-sickness-dubbed-Black-Death-21st-century.html.

3. Katsuo Nishiyama and Jeffrey V. Johnson, "Karoshi—Death from Overwork: Occupational Health Consequences of Japanese Production Management," *International Journal of Health Services* 27, no. 4 (1997), 627–41.

4. Morioka, "Work Till You Drop."

5. Ronald E. Yates, "Japanese Live . . . and Die . . . for Their Work," *Chicago Tribune,* November 13, 1988, http://articles.chicagotribune.com/1988-11-13 /news/8802150740_1_karoshi-japanese-health-and-welfare.

6. Matthew Reiss, "American Karoshi," *New Internationalist* 343 (March 2002).

7. Alina Tugend, "Want to Work Better? Take a Vacation," *New York Times,* June 9, 2008, http://www.nytimes.com/2008/06/09/business/worldbusiness/09iht -vac.4.13584260.html?_r=2.

8. Brooks B. Gump and Karen A. Matthews, "Are Vacations Good for Your Health? The 9-Year Mortality Experience after the Multiple Risk Factor Intervention Trial," *Psychosomatic Medicine* 62, no. 5 (September/October 2000): 608–12.

9. Elaine D. Eaker, Joan Pinsky, and William P. Castelli, "Myocardial Infarction and Coronary Death among Women: Psychosocial Predictors from a 20-Year Fol- low-Up of Women in the Framingham Study," *American Journal of Epidemiology* 135, no. 8 (April 15, 1992): 854–64.

10. S. L. Manne and A. J. Zautra, "Spouse Criticism and Support: Their Association with Coping and Psychological Adjustment among Women with Rheumatoid Arthri- tis," *Journal of Personality and Social Psychology* 56, no. 4 (April 1989): 608–17; Mary C. Davis, Alex J. Zautra, and John W. Reich, "Vulnerability to Stress among Women in Chronic Pain from Fibromyalgia and Osteoarthritis," *Annals of Behavioral Medicine* 23, no. 3 (Summer 2001): 215–26; A. J. Zautra, L. M. John- son, and M. C. Davis, "Positive Affect as a Source of Resilience for Women in Chronic Pain," *Journal of Consulting and Clinical Psychology* 73, no. 2 (April 2005): 212–20.

11. B. A. Huyser and J. C. Parker, "Negative Affect and Pain in Arthritis," *Rheumatic Disease Clinics of North America* 25, no. 1 (February 1999): 105–21; S. A. McLean et al., "Momentary Relationship between Cortisol Secretion and Symptoms in Patients with Fibromyalgia," *Arthritis and Rheumatism* 52, no. 11 (Novem- ber 2005): 3660–69; S. A. McLean et al., "Cerebrospinal Fluid Corticotro- pin-Releasing Factor Concentration Is Associated with Pain but Not Fatigue Symptoms in Patients with Fibromyalgia," *Neuropsychopharmacology* 31, no. 12 (December 2006), 2776–82.

12. L. Bendtsen, "Central and Peripheral Sensitization in Tension-Type Headache," *Current Pain Headache Reports* 7, no. 6 (December 2003): 460–65.

13. Ashley E. Nixon et al., "Can Work Make You Sick? A Meta-Analysis of the Rela- tionships between Job Stressors and Physical Symptoms," *Work & Stress* 25, no. 1 (January–March 2011): 1–22; S. T. Gura, "Yoga for Stress Reduction and Injury Prevention at Work," *Work: Journal of Prevention, Assessment and Rehabilitation* 19, no. 1 (2002): 3–7.

14. R. Rau et al., "Psychosocial Work Characteristics and Perceived Control in Relation to Cardiovascular Rewind at Night," *Journal of Occupational Health Psychology* 6, no. 3 (July 2001): 171–81; K. A. Ertel, K. Karestan, and L. F. Berkman, "Incor- porating Home Demands into Models of Job Strain: Findings from the Work, Family, and Health Network," *Journal of Occupational and Environmental Medicine* 50, no. 11 (November 2008): 1244–52; T. Roth and S. Ancoli-Israel, "Daytime Consequences and Correlates of Insomnia in the United States: Results of the 1991 National Sleep Foundation Survey. II," *Sleep* 22, no. 2 (May 1, 1999):

354–58; M. Jansson and S. J. Linton, "Psychosocial Work Stressors in the Development and Maintenance of Insomnia: A Prospective Study," *Journal of Occupational Health Psychology* 11, no. 3 (July 2006): 241–48.

15. Steven J. Linton and Ing-Liss Bryngelsson, "Insomnia and Its Relationship to Work and Health in a Working-Age Population," *Journal of Occupational Rehabilitation* 10, no. 2 (June 2000): 169–83.

16. G. Aguilera, "Regulation of Pituitary ACTH Secretion during Chronic Stress," *Frontiers in Neuroendocrinology* 15, no. 4 (December 1994): 321–50.

17. A. J. Dittner, S. C. Wessely, and R. G. Brown, "The Assessment of Fatigue: A Practical Guide for Clinicians and Researchers," *Journal of Psychosomatic Research* 56, no. 2 (February 2004): 157–70; Pascal M. L. Franssen et al., "The Association between Chronic Diseases and Fatigue in the Working Population," *Journal of Psychosomatic Research* 54, no. 4 (April 2003): 339–44.

18. Mark A. Demitrack et al., "Evidence for Impaired Activation of the Hypothalamic-Pituitary-Adrenal Axis in Patients with Chronic Fatigue Syndrome," *Journal of Clinical Endocrinology and Metabolism* 73, no. 6 (December 1991): 1224–34.

19. A. K. Smith et al., "Polymorphisms in Genes Regulating the HPA Axis Associated with Empirically Delineated Classes of Unexplained Chronic Fatigue," *Pharmacogenomics* 7, no. 3 (April 2006): 387–94.

20. Jack Sparacino, "Blood Pressure, Stress and Mental Health," *Nursing Research* 31, no. 2 (March–April 1982): 89–94.

21. Nixon et al., "Can Work Make You Sick?"

22. Jay Kandiah, Melissa Yake, and Heather Willett, "Effects of Stress on Eating Practices among Adults," *Family and Consumer Sciences Research Journal* 37, no. 1 (September 2008): 27–38.

23. Ibid.

24. J. Liu et al., "The Melanocortinergic Pathway Is Rapidly Recruited by Acute Emotional Stress and Contributes to Stress-Induced Anorexia and Anxiety-Like Behavior," *Endocrinology* 148, no. 11 (November 2007): 5531–40.

25. Masahiro Ochi et al., "Effect of Chronic Stress on Gastric Emptying and Plasma Ghrelin Levels in Rats," *Life Science* 82, no. 15–16 (April 9, 2008): 862–68.

26. Ricard Farré et al., "Critical Role of Stress in Increased Oesophageal Mucosa Permeability and Dilated Intercellular Spaces," *Gut* 56, no. 9 (February 2007): 1191–97.

27. Martin E. Keck and Florian Holsboer, "Hyperactivity of CRH Neuronal Circuits as a Target for Therapeutic Interventions in Affective Disorders," *Peptides* 22, no. 5 (May 2001): 835–44.

28. T. G. Pickering, "Blood Platelets, Stress, and Cardiovascular Disease," *Psychosomatic Medicine* 55, no. 6 (November/December 1993): 483–84; E. M. Sternberg, "Does Stress Make You Sick and Belief Make You Well? The Science Connecting Body and Mind," *Annals of the New York Academy of Sciences* 917 (January 2000): 1–3.

29. Bert Garssen, "Psychological Factors and Cancer Development: Evidence after 30 Years of Research," *Clinical Psychology Review* 24, no. 3 (July 2004): 315–38; Eric

Raible and Allan S. Jaffe, "Work Stress May Be a Determinant of Coronary Heart Disease," *Cardiology Today* 11, no. 3 (March 2008): 33; S. O. Dalton et al., "Mind and Cancer: Do Psychological Factors Cause Cancer?" *European Journal of Cancer* 38, no. 10 (July 2002): 1313–23; Edna M. V. Reiche, Sandra O. V. Nunes, and Helena K. Morimoto, "Stress, Depression, the Immune System, and Cancer," *Lancet Oncology* 5, no. 10 (October 2004): 617–25; Ljudmila Stojanovich and Dragomir Marisavljevich, "Stress as a Trigger of Autoimmune Disease," *Autoimmunity Reviews* 7, no. 3 (January 2008): 209–13; Eva M. Selhub, "Stress and Distress in Clinical Practice: A Mind-Body Approach," *Nutrition and Clinical Care* 5, no. 4 (July/August 2002): 182–90.

30. Meredith Melnick, "Study: Your Hostile Workplace May Be Killing You," *Time.com,* August 10, 2011, http://healthland.time.com/2011/08/10/study-your-hostile-workplace-may-be-killing-you/.

31. P. Butterworth et al., "The Psychosocial Quality of Work Determines Whether Employment Has Benefits for Mental Health: Results from a Longitudinal National Household Panel Survey," *Occupational and Environmental Medicine* 68, no. 11 (2011): 806–12.

32. Robert Pear, "Gap in Life Expectancy Widens for the Nation," *New York Times,* March 23, 2008, http://www.nytimes.com/2008/03/23/us/23health.html.

33. A. Antonovsky, "Social Class, Life Expectancy, and Overall Mortality," *Milbank Memorial Fund Quarterly* 45, no. 2 (April 1967): 31–73; Raymond Illsley and Deborah Baker, "Contextual Variations in the Meaning of Health Inequality," *Social Science and Medicine* 32, no. 4 (1991): 359–65; Tom Reynolds, "Report Examines Association between Cancer and Socioeconomic Status," *Journal of the National Cancer Institute* 95, no. 19 (2003): 1431–33.

34. "Are Poor People Less Likely to Be Healthy Than Rich People?" Public Health Agency of Canada, September 11, 2008.

35. "Rich People Die Differently," *WebMD,* July 7, 2005, http://men.webmd.com /news/20050707/rich-people-die-differently.

36. Dan Seligman, "Why the Rich Live Longer," *Forbes.com,* June 7, 2004, http://www .forbes.com/forbes/2004/0607/113_print.html.

37. Graham S. Lowe, Grant Schellenberg, and Harry S. Shannon, "Correlates of Employees' Perceptions of a Healthy Work Environment," *American Journal of Health Promotion* 17, no. 6 (July/August 2003): 390–99; Katherine Baicker, David Cutler, and Zirui Song, "Workplace Wellness Programs Can Generate Savings," *Health Affairs* 29, no. 2 (February 2010): 304–11.

38. Beata Tobiasz-Adamczyk and Piotr Brzyski, "Psychosocial Work Conditions as Predictors of Quality of Life at the Beginning of Older Age," *International Journal of Occupational Medicine and Environmental Health* 18, no. 1 (January 2005): 43–52; T. Theorell, "Working Conditions and Health," in *Social Epidemiology,* ed. L. F. Berkman and I. Kawachi (New York: Oxford University Press, 2000), 95–117; E. B. Faragher, M. Cass, and C. L. Cooper, "The Relationship between Job Satisfaction and Health: A Meta-Analysis," *Occupational and Environmental Medicine* 62, no. 2 (February 2005): 105–12; R. Veenhoven, "Healthy Happiness: Effects of Happiness on Physical Health and the Consequences for Preventive Health Care," *Journal of Happiness Studies* 9, no. 3 (September 2008): 449–69; Justina

A. V. Fischer and Alfonso Sousa-Poza, "Does Job Satisfaction Improve the Health of Workers? New Evidence Using Panel Data and Objective Measures of Health," *Health Economics* 18, no. 1 (January 2009): 71–89.

39. Joachim C. Brunstein, "Personal Goals and Subjective Well-Being: A Longitudinal Study," *Journal of Personality and Social Psychology* 65, no. 5 (November 1993): 1061–70.

40. Nancy Cantor, "From Thought to Behavior: 'Having' and 'Doing' in the Study of Personality and Cognition," *American Psychologist* 45, no. 6 (June 1990): 735–50.

41. Tait D. Shanafelt et al., "Career Fit and Burnout among Academic Faculty," *Archives of Internal Medicine* 169, no. 10 (May 25, 2009): 990–95.

42. Amanda Enayati, "A Creative Life Is a Healthy Life," *CNN.com,* May 26, 2012, http://www.cnn.com/2012/05/25/health/enayati-innovation-passion-stress/index.html.

43. Marti Hand, "The Benefits of Integrating Creativity in Healthcare," *Creativity in Healthcare,* accessed May 15, 2012, http://creativityinhealthcare.com/creativity -in-health-caremarti-handarts-in-healthcarehealthcarenursing-3/; Gene D. Cohen et al., "The Impact of Professionally Conducted Cultural Programs on the Physical Health, Mental Health, and Social Functioning of Older Adults," *Gerontologist* 46, no. 6 (2006): 726–34; Daniel A. Monti et al., "A Randomized, Controlled Trial of Mindfulness-Based Art Therapy (MBAT) for Women with Cancer," *Psychooncology* 15, no. 5 (May 2006): 363–73; Bonnie Gabriel et al., "Art Therapy with Adult Bone Marrow Transplant Patients in Isolation: A Pilot Study," *Psychooncology* 10, no. 2 (March/April 2001): 114–13; Joe Verghese et al., "Leisure Activities and the Risk of Dementia in the Elderly," *New England Journal of Medicine* 348 (June 2003): 2508–16; R. F. Cruz and D. L. Sabers, "Dance/Movement Therapy Is More Effective than Previously Reported," *The Arts in Psychotherapy* 25 (1998): 101–104.

Chapter 7

1. Ruut Veenhoven, "World Database of Happiness: Continuous Register of Research on Subjective Appreciation of Life," in *Challenges for Quality of Life in the Contemporary World: Advances in Quality-of-Life Studies, Theory and Research,* ed. W. Glatzer, S. von Below, and M. Stoffregen (Dordrecht, The Netherlands: Kluwer Academic Publishers, 2004).

2. Corey L. M. Keyes, "Mental Illness and/or Mental Health? Investigating Axioms of the Complete State Model of Health," *Journal of Consulting and Clinical Psychology* 73, no. 3 (Jun 2005): 539–48.

3. Thomson Healthcare, Washington, D.C. "Ranking America's Mental Health: An Analysis of Depression across the States," *Mental Health America,* December 11, 2007, http://www.mentalhealthamerica.net/go/state-ranking.

4. National Institute of Mental Health, "Any Mood Disorder Among Adults," accessed May 15, 2012, https://www.nimh.nih.gov/health/statistics/any-mood-disorder.shtml.

5. Charles Eisenstein, "Mutiny of the Soul," CharlesEisenstein.org, October 2008, https://charleseisenstein.org/essays/mutiny/.

6. R. Veenhoven, *Conditions of Happiness* (Dordrecht, The Netherlands: Kluwer Academic Publishers, 1984).

7. Yoichi Chida and Andrew Steptoe. "Positive Psychological Well-Being and Mortality: A Quantitative Review of Prospective Observational Studies," *Psychosomatic Medicine* 70, no. 7 (September 2008): 741–56.

8. Michael Lemonick, "The Biology of Joy," *Time,* January 9, 2005.

9. Joshua Wolf Shenk, "What Makes Us Happy?" *Atlantic,* January 2009, http://www.theatlantic.com/magazine/archive/2009/06/what–makes–us–happy/7439/#.

10. Bernie S. Siegel, *Love, Medicine & Miracles* (New York: Harper & Row, 1986), 76.

11. Christopher Peterson, Martin E. Seligman, and George E. Vaillant, "Pessimistic Explanatory Style Is a Risk Factor for Physical Illness: A Thirty-Five-Year Longitudinal Study," *Journal of Personality and Social Psychology* 55, no. 1 (July 1988): 23–27.

12. Lisa G. Aspinwall and Richard G. Tedeschi, "The Value of Positive Psychology for Health Psychology: Progress and Pitfalls in Examining the Relation of Positive Phenomena to Health," *Annals of Behavioral Medicine* 39, no. 1 (February 2010): 4–15.

13. Erik J. Giltay et al., "Dispositional Optimism and All-Cause and Cardiovascular Mortality in a Prospective Cohort of Elderly Dutch Men and Women," *Archives of General Psychiatry* 61, no. 11 (November 2004): 1126–35.

14. Sheldon Cohen et al., "Positive Emotional Style Predicts Resistance to Illness after Experimental Exposure to Rhinovirus or Influenza A Virus," *Psychosomatic Medicine* 68, no. 6 (November 1, 2006): 809–15.

15. Michael Lemonick, "The Biology of Joy."

16. Martin Seligman, *Learned Optimism: How to Change Your Mind and Your Life* (New York: Vintage Books, 1991).

17. Christopher Peterson and Mechele E. De Avila, "Optimistic Explanatory Style and the Perception of Health Problems," *Journal of Clinical Psychology* 51, no. 1 (January 1995): 128–32; Kymberley K. Bennett and Marta Elliott, "Pessimistic Explanatory Style and Cardiac Health: What Is the Relation and the Mechanism that Links Them?" *Basic and Applied Social Psychology* 27, no. 3 (September 2005): 239–48; Katri Räikkönen et al., "Effects of Optimism, Pessimism, and Trait Anxiety on Ambulatory Blood Pressure and Mood During Everyday Life," *Journal of Personality and Social Psychology* 76, no. 1 (January 1999): 104–13.

18. Christopher Peterson, "Explanatory Style as a Risk Factor for Illness," *Cognitive Therapy and Research* 12, no. 2 (1988): 119–32.

19. Laura D. Kubzansky and Rebecca C. Thurston, "Emotional Vitality and Incident Coronary Heart Disease: Benefits of Healthy Psychological Functioning," *Archives of General Psychiatry* 64, no. 12 (December 2007): 1393–1401.

20. Shelley E. Taylor et al., "Are Self-Enhancing Cognitions Associated with Healthy or Unhealthy Biological Profiles?" *Journal of Personality and Social Psychology* 85, no. 4 (October 2003): 605–15.

21. Christopher Peterson and Martin E. Seligman, "Causal Explanations as a Risk Factor for Depression: Theory and Evidence," *Psychological Review* 91 no. 3 (July 1984): 347–74.

22. Chida and Steptoe, "Positive Psychological Well-Being and Mortality."

23. M. A. Visintainer, J. R. Volpicelli, and M. E. Seligman, "Tumor Rejection in Rats after Inescapable or Escapable Shock," *Science* 216, no. 4544 (April 23, 1982): 437–39.

24. M. Seligman and M. Visintainer, "Tumor Rejection and Early Experience of Uncontrollable Shock in the Rat," in *Affect, Conditioning, and Cognition: Essays on the Determinants of Behavior*, ed. F. R. Brush and J. B. Overmier (Hillsdale, NJ: Erlbaum, 1985), 203–5.

25. Ellen J. Langer and Judith Rodin, "Effects of Choice and Enhanced Personal Responsibility for the Aged: A Field Experiment in an Institutional Setting," *Journal of Personality and Social Psychology* 34, no. 2 (1976): 191–98.

26. Martin Seligman, *Authentic Happiness: Using the New Positive Psychology to Realize Your Potential for Lasting Fulfillment* (New York: Free Press, 2003).

27. Deborah D. Danner, David A. Snowdon, and Wallace V. Friesen, "Positive Emotions in Early Life and Longevity: Findings from the Nun Study," *Journal of Personality and Social Psychology* 80, no. 5 (May 2001): 804–13.

28. R. Veenhoven, "Healthy Happiness: Effects of Happiness on Physical Health and the Consequences for Preventive Health Care," *Journal of Happiness Studies* 9, no. 3 (September 2008): 449–69.

29. Janice K. Kiecolt-Glaser et al., "Hostile Marital Interactions, Proinflammatory Cytokine Production, and Wound Healing," *Archives of General Psychiatry* 62, no. 12 (December 2005): 1377–84; Janice K. Kiecolt-Glaser et al., "Emotions, Morbidity, and Mortality: New Perspectives from Psychoneuroimmunology," *Annual Review of Psychology* 53 (February 2002): 83–107.

30. J. Licinio, P. W. Gold, and M. L. Wong, "A Molecular Mechanism for Stress-Induced Alterations in Susceptibility to Disease," *Lancet* 346, no. 8967 (July 1995): 104–6; Ryan T. Howell, Margaret L. Kern, and Sonja Lyubomirsky, "Health Benefits: Meta-Analytically Determining the Impact of Well-Being on Objective Health Outcomes," *Health Psychology Review* 1, no. 1 (July 2007): 83–136.

31. Michael Lemonick, "The Biology of Joy," 2005; Erin S. Costanzo et al., "Mood and Cytokine Response to Influenza Virus in Older Adults," *Journals of Gerontology* 59, no. 12 (December 2004): 1328–33; Marian L. Kohut et al., "Exercise and Psychosocial Factors Modulate Immunity to Influenza Vaccine in Elderly Individuals," *Journals of Gerontology* 57, no. 9 (September 2002): 557–62.

32. R. W. Bartrop et al., "Depressed Lymphocyte Function after Bereavement," *Lancet* 1, no. 8016 (April 16, 1977): 834–36.

33. D. M. Byrnes et al., "Stressful Events, Pessimism, Natural Killer Cell Cytotoxicity, and Cytotoxic/Suppressor T Cells in HIV+ Black Women at Risk for Cervical Cancer," *Psychosomatic Medicine* 60, no. 6 (November/December 1998): 714–22.

34. Peter Kirsch et al., "Oxytocin Modulates Neural Circuitry for Social Cognition and Fear in Humans," *Journal of Neuroscience* 25, no. 49 (December 7, 2005): 11489–93; C. Sue Carter, "Neuroendocrine Perspectives on Social Attachment and Love," *Psychoneuroendocrinology* 23, no. 8 (November 1998): 779–818.

35. Tiina-Mari Lyyra, "Predictors of Mortality in Old Age: Contribution of Self-Rated Health, Physical Functions, Life Satisfaction and Social Support on Survival among Older People," *University of Jyväskylä: Studies in Sport, Physical Education and Health* 119 (2006).

36. Ed Diener and Micaela Chan, "Happy People Live Longer: Subjective Well-Being Contributes to Health and Longevity," *Applied Psychology: Health and Well-Being* 3, no. 1 (March 2011); Lemonick, "The Biology of Joy"; Chida and Steptoe, "Positive Psychological Well-Being and Mortality."

37. S. Levy et al., "Survival Hazards Analysis in First Recurrent Breast Cancer Patients: Seven Year Follow Up," *Psychosomatic Medicine* 50, no. 5 (September/October 1988): 520–28.

38. Veenhoven, "Healthy Happiness"; Leonard R. Derogatis, Martin D. Abeloff, and Nick Melisaratos, "Psychological Coping Mechanisms and Survival Time in Metastatic Breast Cancer," *Journal of the American Medical Association* 242, no. 14 (October 5, 1979): 1504–8.

39. Frits Van Dam, "Does Happiness Heal," in *How Harmful Is Happiness? Consequences of Enjoying Life or Not,* ed. R. Veenhoven (The Netherlands: Universitaire Pers Rotterdam, 1989), 17–23.

40. Richard E. Lucas et al., "Reexamining Adaptation and the Set Point Model of Happiness: Reactions to Changes in Marital Status," *Journal of Personality and Social Psychology* 84, no. 3 (March 2003): 527–39.

41. Sonja Lyubomirsky, Kennon M. Sheldon, and David Schkade, "Pursuing Happiness: The Architecture of Sustainable Change," *Review of General Psychology* 9, no. 2 (June 2005): 111–31.

42. Andrew M. Greeley, *Ecstasy: A Way of Knowing* (New Jersey: Prentice Hall, 1974).

43. S. W. Cole et al., "Accelerated Course of Human Immunodeficiency Virus Infection in Gay Men Who Conceal Their Homosexual Identity," *Psychosomatic Medicine* 58, no. 3 (May/June 1996): 219–31.

Chapter 8

1. "Easy Ways to Take the Edge Off," *ABC News Video,* April 22, 2009, http://abcnews .go.com/video/playerIndex?id=7392433.

2. Razali Salleh Mohd, "Life Event, Stress and Illness," *Malaysian Journal of Medical Sciences* 15, no. 4 (October 2008): 9–18, https://www.ncbi.nlm.nih.gov/pmc/ articles/PMC3341916/.

3. "Eliciting the Relaxation Response," Benson-Henry Institute for Mind Body Medicine, Massachusetts General Hospital, accessed May 15, 2012, http://www .massgeneral.org/bhi/basics/eliciting_rr.aspx.

4. Richard J. Davidson et al., "Alterations in Brain and Immune Function Produced by Mindfulness Meditation," *Psychosomatic Medicine* 65, no. 4 (July/August 2003): 564–70.

5. Bonnie Horrigan, "Meditation Reduces Pain Scores," *Explore: The Journal of Science and Healing* 7, no. 4 (July/August 2011): 215–16; R. Manocha et al., "A Randomized, Controlled Trial of Meditation for Work Stress, Anxiety and Depressed Mood in Full-Time Workers," *Evidence-Based Complementary and Alternative Medicine* (June 7, 2011); W. P. Smith, W. C. Compton, and W. B. West, "Meditation as an Adjunct to a Happiness Enhancement Program," *Journal of Clinical Psychology* 51, no. 2 (March 1995): 269–73; A. Nesvold et al., "Increased Heart Rate Variability during Nondirective Meditation," *European Journal of Preventive Cardiology* 19, no. 4 (August 2012): 773–80; F. Zeidan et al., "Mindfulness Meditation Improves Cognition: Evidence of Brief Mental Training," *Consciousness and Cognition* 19, no. 2 (June 10, 2010): 597–605; L. Fortney and M. Taylor, "Meditation in Medical Practice: A Review of the Evidence and Practice," *Primary Care* 37, no. 1 (March 2010): 81–90; R. Walsh and S. L. Shapiro, "The Meeting of Meditative Disciplines and Western Psychology: A Mutually Enriching Dialogue," *American Psychologist* 61, no. 3 (April 2006): 227–39; Maura Paul-Labrador et al., "Effects of a Randomized Controlled Trial of Transcendental Meditation on Components of the Metabolic Syndrome in Subjects with Coronary Heart Disease," *Archives of Internal Medicine* 166, no. 11 (June 12, 2006): 1218–24; S. I. Nidich et al., "A Randomized Controlled Trial of the Effects of Transcendental Meditation on Quality of Life in Older Breast Cancer Patients," *Integrative Cancer Therapy* 8, no. 3 (September 2009): 228–34.

6. American Psychological Association, "Stress in America Press Room," http://apa.org/news/press/releases/stress/index.aspx.

7. "Almost a Quarter of All Disease Caused by Environmental Exposure," World Health Organization, June 16, 2006, http://www.who.int/mediacentre/news/releases/2006/pr32/en/index.html.

Chapter 9

1. Adler, A. D., Strunk, D. R., & Fazio. R. H. (2015). What changes in cognitive therapy for depression? An examination of cognitive therapy skills and maladaptive beliefs. *Behavior Therapy*, 46, 96–109.

2. https://www.eftuniverse.com/research-studies/eft-research

3. https://www.energypsych.org/page/Research_Landing

4. A. J. Cunningham et al., "Fighting for Life: A Qualitative Analysis of the Process of Psychotherapy-Assisted Self-Help in Patients with Metastatic Cancer," *Integrative Cancer Therapies*, 1, no. 2 (June 2002): 146–61.

5. https://www.ncbi.nlm.nih.gov/pmc/articles/PMC5724984/

6. S. L. Shapiro, "Spontaneous Regression of Cancer," *Eye, Ear, Nose, Throat Monthly*, 46, No. 10 (October 1967): 1306–10.

7. S. A. Cann et al., "Spontaneous Regression of Pancreatic Cancer," *Case Reports & Clinical Practice Review*, 9 (July 2004): 293–96.

INDEX

C

Cacioppo, John, 105, 106
Cain, Susan, 109
Callings, 21–22, 100, 126, 129–130
CAM (complementary and alternative
     medicine) treatments, 50, 65–66, 68
Cancer, 102–103
Cannon, Walter, 15, 167
CBT (Cognitive Behavioral Therapy),
     199–200
Cellular environment, 32–34
Cheerfulness, 52, 146–148, 152–153
Chicago Tribune, 115
Childhood
     negative expectations programming
          during, 30, 34–36, 38–40
     traumas of, 102–104, 106
Chinese Americans, 23–24
Chronic diseases
     depression and, 137
     emotional health and, 136, 137,
          138–139, 152–153
     loneliness and, 105
     medical hexing and, 41
     pre- and perinatal influences on,
          34–35
     stress response and, 168
     work stress and, 114–117, 122–123
Church. *See* Spirituality
Church, Dawson, 159, 160, 161–162,
     174
Classical conditioning, 12
Clinton, Asha, 30–31, 200
Cognitive Behavioral Therapy (CBT),
     199–200
Cohen, Sanford, 28
Cole, Steve, 162–163
Cole, Warren, 19
Collaborating among health-care
     providers, 67–68, 193, 211–218, 244
College student study, on happiness,
     136–137, 138
Community. *See* Interpersonal health
Complementary and alternative
     medicine (CAM) treatments, 50,
     65–66, 68
Conditioning, 12
Consequences, of ABC method,
     154–156
Control, being in (empowerment), 118,
     138, 144, 145–146. *See also* Inner
     Pilot Light

Cooling practices, of meditation,
     172–173
Corticotropin-releasing hormone
     (CRH), 82, 106, 122
Cortisol
     about, 82–84
     anxiety and, 149
     creative expression and, 128
     depression and, 149
     happiness and, 151
     loneliness and, 105–106
     meditation and, 171
     self-esteem and, 139
     stress response and, 15
     work stress and, 120–122
Coupled relationships, 97, 101–104,
     177. *See also* Interpersonal health
Cousins, Norman, 64, 66
Creative expression
     defined, 127
     interpersonal health and, 111–112
     overview, 76–79, 88
     relaxation response and, 127–128,
          177
     self-diagnosis exercise for, 232
     work/life purpose and, 127–129
CRH (corticotropin-releasing
     hormone), 82, 106, 122
Cultural beliefs, 53, 55–56
Cunningham, Alistair, 249–250
Cured (Rediger), 20
The Cure Within (Harrington), xxv
Curing and healing disease. *See also*
     Spontaneous remissions
     cured, defined, 186
     emotional health and, 152–153
     healed, but not cured, 186–187,
          251–252
     healed and cured, 186–187, 252–254
     medical hexing and, 41
     placebo effect and, 17–18
     symptom relief versus, 17–18
Cutting for Stone (Verghese), 255

D

The Daily Flame (Rankin), 224
Dalai Lama, 133, 167
Default mode network (DMN), 159,
     172
Delivery, of diagnoses and prognoses,
     42–43, 60–62

G

Gastrointestinal distress, 122
Genetic determinism (gene myopia),
   29–30, 32, 35
Ghrelin, 121–122
The Gifts of Imperfection (Brown), 110
Gita, Bhagavad, 113
Gladwell, Malcolm, 93
God Box Meditation, 207–211, 244
"Good" versus "bad genes," 32
Gøtzsche, Peter, 13–14
Grant Study, 136–137, 138
Gratitude
   for financial health, 78
   happiness and, 158
   meditations on, 175–176
   for self-healing, 246
   Whole Health Cairn wellness model
      on, 88
   for work/life purpose, 130
Greater Than the Sum of Our Parts
   (Schwartz), 243
Greeley, Andrew, 161–162
Guilt, 101, 110, 220

H

Hand, Marti, 128
Happiness. *See also* Emotional and
   mental health
   defined, 135, 151
   Grant Study on, 136–137, 138
   immune system and, 150
   interpersonal health and, 158, 159
   overview, 133–134, 135–136
   physiology of, 150–152, 158–159
   prescription for, 157–163
   spirituality and, 99–100
   work/life purpose and, 125–129
Harrington, Anne, xxv
Harvard student study, on happiness,
   136–137, 138
Harvey, Andrew, 165
Headaches, 120
Heal At Last (organization), 216–217,
   244
Healing, curing disease versus. *See*
   Curing and healing disease
Healing environments, 76–79, 88, 181,
   234–235

Healing round table, 67–68, 193, 211–
   218, 244
Health beliefs
   CAM treatments and, 65–66
   conditioning and, 12
   delivery of medical information and,
      42–43, 60–62
   exercise for examining, 198–200,
      243
   expectations and. *See* Negative
      expectations; Positive
      expectations
   of health-care provider and health
      outcomes, 51–54
   immune system affected by, 16
   mechanism of, 56–57
   as placebo effect, 65–66
   power of, 45–49
   ritual of treatment, 12–13, 15, 16,
      55–56
   spontaneous remissions and, 13–14,
      18–22
   symptom perception, 18
Health-care providers
   collaboration among, 67–68, 193,
      211–218, 244
   delivery of diagnoses and prognoses
      by, 42–43, 60–62
   guidelines for discerning Six Step
      candidates, 247–251
   mind-body connection pioneers,
      xxiv–xxvi
   mission of, 80–81
   negative expectations of, 52
   nurturing care for, 63–64
   patients' expectations of, 47–49
   positive expectations of, 51–54
   trust in, 52–53
Healthy relationships. *See* Interpersonal
   health
Heartburn, 122
HeartMath practice, 175
Heart rate variability, 84–85
Hedonistic adaptation, 158
Helplessness (learned), 123–125, 142–
   146, 150, 152
Hemispheric synchronization, 174
Hemi-Sync meditations, 174
Hippocampus, 149, 159–160
Hiraoka, Satoru, 114–115
Hirshberg, Caryle, 19
Hmong culture, 55–56
Hope. *See* Positive expectations

The How of Happiness (Lyubomirsky), 125, 158
Hróbjartsson, Asbjørn, 13–14
Hyperventilation, 121
Hypothalamic-pituitary-adrenal (HPA) axis, 15, 29, 82, 106, 119–120, 151
Hypothalamus, 82–84, 106, 151, 166. *See also* Dopamine

I

IFS (Internal Family Systems) model, 37–38, 160–161, 174, 189, 224–227
Immune system
    emotional health and, 138–139, 150
    health beliefs' effect on, 16
    learned helplessness and, 143–145
    loneliness and, 105, 106
    mind-body connection and, 170–171
    placebo effect and, 16, 17
    psychoneuroimmunology on, 170–171
    stress response and, 83
Infertility, 207–208
Information Age, 116
Inner Pilot Light
    connecting and surrendering to, 192–193, 203–211, 244
    description of, 87–88, 205
    as Prescription writing guide, 194–195
    reunion of conscious and unconscious mind through, 190–191
    self-diagnosis and, 224, 229–230
Inside Out (film), 37
Internal Family Systems (IFS) model, 37–38, 160–161, 174, 189, 224–227
International Labour Organization, 117
Interpersonal health, 91–112
    coupled relationships, 97, 101–104, 177
    creative expression and, 128
    happiness and, 158, 159
    life expectancy and, 96–99, 101, 105
    loneliness and, 104–107, 111–112. *See also* Loneliness
    negative relationship dynamics and, 102–103, 107–109
    overview, 76–79, 88, 91–95
    physiology of, 84–85, 104–107, 159

relaxation response and, 177
Roseto example, 91–95
self-diagnosis exercise for, 230–231
spiritual community, 98–101
stress response and, 95, 96–106, 108
supportive community as preventive medicine, 91–96, 103
vagus nerve and, 84–85
vulnerability and, 109–111
Introverts, 106, 109, 193
Isolation. *See* Loneliness
Italian Americans, 91–95

J

Japan, work/life balance in, 114–115
Jones, Jonathan, 48–49
The Journal of Clinical Investigation, 4–5
Journal of Clinical Oncology, 97
Journal of Epidemiology and Community Health, 101
Journal of the American Medical Association, 7

K

Kaptchuk, Ted, 12–13, 14, 18, 50–51, 55, 65
Karoshi, 114–117
Katie, Byron, 199
Kennedy, John F., 137
Kigyo-senchi, 114–115
Klopfer, Bruno, 3–4
Kornfield, Jack, 174
Kubzansky, Laura, 139

L

Landy, John, 196
Learned helplessness, 123–125, 142–146, 150, 152
Learned optimism, 156
Learned Optimism (Seligman), 154–156
Lee, Hmong shaman Va Meng, 55
Life expectancy
    depression and, 137
    emotional health and, 137, 138–139, 146–148, 162–163
    financial health and, 123–124

Negative relationship dynamics, 102–
  103, 107–109
New England Journal of Medicine, 5–6,
  13–14, 50–51, 52
New Scientist, 97–98
New York Times, xxi, 55–56
Nitric oxide, 89, 150, 152
Nocebo effect, 25–30, 34, 36, 40, 52–53
Non-local mind, 206
Norepinephrine, 83, 106, 149–150
Northrup, Christiane, 221
Novack, Nancy, 45–46
Nucleus accumbens, 16–17, 151–152
Nuns, 146–148
Nurturing care
  CAM treatments as, 50, 65–66
  harm from absence of, 57–59
  for health-care providers, 63–64
  health-care providers' beliefs and,
    51–54
  as heart of medicine, 46, 55–56, 59,
    64, 67–69
  physiological responses to, 56–57
  placebo effect and, 9, 13, 16, 49–56,
    65–66
  relaxation response to, 46, 56–57
  self-healing of body and, 56–57

O

Oliver, Mary, 129
One Mind, 206
O'Payne, Cecilia, 147–148
Optimism
  gratitude and, 88
  happiness and, 158
  healing power of, 139–142, 153
  learned helplessness and, 142–143,
    145, 152
  learned optimism, 156
  life expectancy and, 138–139
  overview, 133, 135–136
  patient outcomes and, 52
  permanency of trauma and, 137–138
  radical remissions and, 246
O'Regan, Brendan, 19
Orthodox Jews, 98
Outliers (Gladwell), 93
Oxytocin, 33, 89, 108, 150–152

P

Parasympathetic system, 15–16, 34,
  83–84, 128, 171, 177–178
Pasternak, Boris, 73
Patient intake forms, new approach to,
  xxxiii–xxxv
*The Pavlovian Journal of Biological
  Science*, 26
Peabody, Francis, 45
Perinatal developmental influences, 35
Personal responsibility, 221
Pert, Candace, 170–171
Pessimism
  immune system and, 150
  learned helplessness and, 142–143,
    145, 152
  life expectancy and, 138–139
  permanency of trauma and, 137–138
  prescription for, 154–156
Peterson, Chris, 138
Petri dish stem cell experiment, 32–33
Physical health
  overview, 76–79, 88
  self-diagnosis exercise for, 235–236
Pituitary gland, 82, 106, 151–152
Placebo effect, 3–22
  in CAM treatments, 65–66
  case studies, 3–5
  defined, 14
  immune system and, 16, 17
  mind-body connection and, 34
  nurturing care and, 49–56, 65–66
  physiological responses to, 10–11,
    12, 14–17, 18, 34
  placebo, defined, 6
  positive expectations and, 8–9, 12,
    15, 16–17
  power of, 6–7
  relaxation response and, 168
  as remembered wellness, 168
  ritual of treatment and, 49–51
  spontaneous remissions and, 13–14,
    18–22
  studies on, 5–6, 8–9, 13–14, 15, 16
  susceptibility to, 10
  symptom relief versus curing
    disease, 17–18
  traditional explanations for, 11–14
Plath, Sylvia, 91
Polyvagal Theory, 84
Porges, Stephen, 84
Positive expectations

Q

R

S

manifestation as physical symptoms, 15
to negative expectations, 29, 30, 34, 36–37, 40–43
nurturing care and, 56–57
physiology of, 15, 29, 81–85, 96
purpose of, 82
repetitive, 81–85
self-diagnosis of, 219–221
to sex, 83, 103–104
to spirituality, 101
subconscious mind and, 36
symptoms of, 119–122, 223–225
to traumas, 103, 105
work-related, 117–125
Subconscious mind
childhood programming of, 30, 34–36, 38–40
creative expression and, 128
illnesses as protection belief, 189–191
negative core beliefs of, 35–40
positive expectations and, 36
reprogramming of, 40
Supportive community. *See* Heal At Last; Healing round table; Interpersonal health
Sympathetic nervous system, 15, 82–84, 106, 121–122

T

Tajiri, Shunichiro, 115
Tapping, 200
Thomas, K. B., 52, 55
Thought-stopping technique, 155
Tibetan monks, 167
Timeless Healing (Benson), 170
Transcendental Meditation (TM), 166, 169
Traumas
anxiety and, 149
from childhood, 102–104, 106
epigenetics and, 31–32
loneliness and, 104, 106–107, 109
meditation for moving past, 177–178
meditation resistance and, 176–177
negative core beliefs and, 30–31, 37–38
negative relationship dynamics, 102–103, 107–109

permanency of, 137–139
pessimism and, 156
physiology of, 149
providers for addressing, 187–188
as root cause of illness, 194
sexuality and, 103–104
spiritual, 204
stress response to, 103, 105
The Treatment of Multiple Personality Disorder, 26–27
Trine, Ralph Waldo, 23
Trivers, Robert, 16
Trust, in health-care providers, 52–53
Turner, Kelly, 20, 21, 100, 248, 259–260
29 Gifts (Walker), 88–89
Twin studies, 157

U

United States, work/life balance in, 116–117
An Untethered Soul (Singer), 206

V

Vacation time, 116
Vagus nerve, 83–85, 107
Verghese, Abraham, 255
Visintainer, Madelon, 143–144
"Voodoo death," 27–28, 29
Vulnerability, 109–111, 209

W

Walker, Cami, 88–89
Wallace, Robert Keith, 166
Warming practices, of meditation, 172–173
"Washout phase," 9
Weight loss and gain, 121–122
Weil, Andrew, 41
Wellness, sickness versus, 79–81
West, Philip, 3–4
When the Body Says No (Maté), 108
White coat hypertension, 165
Whole Health Cairn wellness model, 73–89
components of, 85–89
contributing factors to, 76–79, 88.

See also Creative expression;
Emotional and mental health;
Financial health; Healing
environments; Interpersonal
health; Physical health; Sexuality;
Spirituality; Work/life purpose
for diagnosing root cause of illness,
193–194, 218–237
overview, 73–76
The Prescription and, 236–238
sickness versus wellness, 79–81
Whole Health Medicine Institute, 59,
61–62, 68, 185, 215
Witness consciousness, 172
Wolf, Stewart, 92–95
Workaholics Anonymous, 117
Work/life purpose, 113–131
balance between work and life,
226–228
chronic diseases and, 114–117,
122–123
creative expression and, 127–129
death by overwork, 114–117
defined, 126
financial health and, 123–125
finding your calling, 126, 129–130
happiness and, 125–129
job stress, symptoms of, 119–122
life expectancy and, 114–117,
123–124
overview, 76–79, 88, 113–114
self-diagnosis exercise for, 231–232
vacation time, 116
work stress, prescription for,
130–131
work stress, types of, 117–119
Wright, Mr., 3–4

Y

Yoga practice, 175–176

ACKNOWLEDGMENTS

Writing a book is like giving birth. You might have to go through labor and do the pushing, but it takes a whole team of midwives to support you through the gestation and usher your baby out into the world. I have been blessed with dozens of midwives, and to those who supported my process through both editions of this book, I am infinitely grateful.

First, I have to thank every brave, badass soul who ever dared to work through the Six Steps to Healing Yourself as part of your healing journey. Had you all not embraced this work, passed it on to friends, shouted it from the rooftops on your blogs, marked it up and passed it to your loved ones, given it to your clients and patients, and bought it for those who get labeled with scary diagnoses, I never would have had the chance to write a revised edition of this book if you hadn't made this book an international bestseller. I hope this revised edition helps you take your journey even deeper. All of us together are changing the face of medicine.

My deepest thanks go to my mentor Rachel Naomi Remen, M.D., who scraped me off the floor 12 years ago when I was at professional rock bottom, plopped me in a circle of loving doctors who loved me back to life, and said, "Don't join something; build something." Were it not for your influence in my life and in the world of mind-body medicine, this book would never exist. I bow before you with my whole heart. Knowing you has fundamentally transformed me in ways I will never be able to explain or repay. I know you will not be with me forever, and this awareness is with me every day. As Jeff Foster says, "Right now, we stand on sacred and holy ground, for that which will be lost has not yet been lost, and realizing this is the key to unspeakable joy." Unspeakable joy says it all. I love you, Rachel.

To Asha Clinton, Ph.D., my personal therapist and the founder of Advanced Integrative Therapy (AIT), whose practices have changed not only my point of view about healing but have helped me heal my own trauma so I can help others heal theirs, you are a gift. Thank you for giving me a chance to move beyond my wounding into a more authentic, emotionally attuned, broken open heart.

My gratitude to my literary agent, Michele Martin, who invited me to write the one book I could spend the rest of my life shouting from the rooftops, goes beyond words. There have been many more books since this one, and my heartfelt awe over how blessed I am to have you as my agent leaves me bowing on my knees now more than ever. This book is as much yours as mine. Thank you for being my ally in every possible way.

To my editor Anne Barthel who helped me nail down the ineffable in this second edition, your patience with my process astounds me. Bless you! To Reid Tracy, the late Louise Hay, Patty Gift, Sally Mason, and the rest of the team at Hay House who helped me birth the first edition, I am so grateful you took a chance on me.

To my daughter, Siena Klein, thank you for helping me learn how to make motherhood my number one priority while still fulfilling my calling in the world. You are such a part of why this book matters to me. May the future of medicine you inhabit reflect the changes we're trying to make in the world. I love you and am so grateful you chose me as your mother. Your radiant presence in my life is one of the greatest blessings I could ever hope to experience.

To April French, my "home tree," thank you for holding the balloon string of my floating visions for so many years. I will never be able to say thank you enough.

To Pearl Macalley, who miraculously managed to turn three people's jobs into one she excels at beyond measure, you are my professional rock. Thank you for anchoring my work on the web.

To my bestie Diane Hunter, how can I say thank you enough for being a sounding board as I wrestled with this material for so many years? It is with the full waterfall of my heart pouring over you that I offer you my heartfelt gratitude. Your presence in my life makes so much of this work possible.

To my brother Chris and my sister Keli who have walked with me through losing both of our parents, thank you for your steadfastness. As the surviving Rankins from our clan, I hope what's in this book will help us all live a life span that equals our health span so we can be here for our kids as they grow up so quickly.

To my aunt Trudy Rankin, who introduced me to the field of mind-body medicine long before I was ready to get curious about it, bless you for your patience and your influence.

A huge thank-you to Tricia Barrett for helping me compose the self-inquiry questions in Step Four. Your intuitive gifts and ability to tap into collective consciousness made that section so much richer.

To the pioneering faculty of the Whole Health Medicine Institute, who have helped me take the work of Mind Over Medicine and train doctors, therapists, and healers who are facilitating the Six Steps to Healing Yourself with patients all over the world, I cannot thank you enough for believing in me, this work, and the mission we all serve together. So many thanks to all of you: Bernie Siegel, M.D., Rachel N. Remen, M.D., Gabor Maté, M.D., Joan Borysenko, Ph.D., Bruce H. Lipton, Ph.D., Larry Dossey, M.D., Christiane Northrup, M.D., Steve Sisgold, Neha Sangwan, M.D., Sara Gottfried, M.D., Donna Eden, Dawson Church, Ph.D., William Bengston, Ph.D., Asha Clinton, Ph.D., Richard Schwartz, Ph.D., Kelly Turner, Ph.D., Sue Morter, SARK, Rachel Carlton Abrams, M.D., Alberto Villoldo, Ph.D., Tosha Silver, Robert Augustus Masters, Ph.D., Pamela Wible, M.D., James Maskell, Brandy Gillmore, Ph.D., Mary Louder, M.D., Kay Corpus, M.D., Bruce Cryer, Eric Pearl, Jillian Fleer, Cynthia Li, M.D., Roger Walsh, Ph.D., Shamini Jain, Ph.D., Thomas Hübl, Starla Fitch, M.D., Shiloh Sophia, Lynne McTaggart, Jeffrey Rediger, M.D., and Christine Gibson, M.D.

Thank you also to those who came before me, whose research and contributions to this field of medicine influenced this book: Dean Ornish, Andrew Weil, Anne Harrington, Ted Kaptchuk, Fabrizio Benedetti, Norman Cousins, Walter Cannon, Herbert Benson, Arnold Hutschnecker, Martin Seligman, Sonja Lyubomirsky, Brené Brown, and so many more.

So many thanks to all the students and graduates of the Whole Health Medicine Institute, the consciousness and healing training program for health care providers and healers who care about spreading this work and bringing it to those who are ready for it, we couldn't do what we're doing to heal health care if we weren't all in this together. It takes a village, and you all rock my world.

To Kira Siebert, Tara Carnegie, Matt Singmin, Sheila Klink, and everyone else who is helping me birth the Heal At Last project as a way to bring this work to those who might not otherwise be able to access it, thank you for trusting me and visioning with me. May our bold vision to bring these healing circles to anyone who is ready to dive deep one day be realized.

A giant thank-you to all the people at the Institute of Noetic Sciences for all the work you put into studying how the mind can heal the body. Your Spontaneous Remission Project was a godsend, and your friendship and professional support over the years is so appreciated.

To Katsy, Emma, Brandy, Mary, Sweigh, Charles, Maja, Matt, Monique, Christine, Maya, Ed, Amanda, Jonathan, Nick, Tiffany, Saida, Del, Kristen, Annie, and Luke, just because you're all so precious to me and I couldn't have done this without you.

ABOUT THE AUTHOR

Lissa Rankin, M.D., is a physician, the *New York Times* best-selling author of six books, a researcher of the phenomenon of "spontaneous" remission, an expert in the intersection of science and the sacred, and the founder of the Whole Health Medicine Institute, a transformational training program focusing on consciousness and healing for health-care providers and healers. The last seven years, she adventured around the globe researching *Sacred Medicine*, the follow-up to *Mind Over Medicine*. This journey down the rabbit hole led her to study with shamans in Peru, qigong masters from China, Balinese healers, Native American medicine men and women, Hawaiian kahunas, mind-body medicine doctors, and energy healers, trauma therapists, and biofield scientists in her home country. Dr. Rankin's passion for self-healing led to two national public television specials, four TEDx talks that have been viewed over five million times, and an online community of people practicing the Six Steps to Healing Yourself at HealingSoulTribe.com. She leads workshops, both online and at retreat centers like Esalen, 1440, Omega, and Kripalu. Her latest philanthropic social justice project, Heal At Last, is committed to eliminating the public health epidemic of loneliness while bringing cutting-edge healing modalities to anyone who feels ready to do this deep inner work, regardless of socioeconomic status, race, or gender identity. Learn more about Dr. Rankin's work at LissaRankin.com and HealAtLast.org. You can also follow her on Facebook, Twitter, and Instagram.

Hay House Titles of Related Interest

YOU CAN HEAL YOUR LIFE, the movie,
starring Louise Hay & Friends
(available as an online streaming video)
www.hayhouse.com/louise-movie

THE SHIFT, the movie,
starring Dr. Wayne W. Dyer
(available as an online streaming video)
www.hayhouse.com/the-shift-movie

***

BLISS BRAIN: The Neuroscience of Remodeling Your Brain for Resilience, Creativity, and Joy, by Dawson Church

MIND TO MATTER: The Astonishing Science of How Your Brain Creates Material Reality, by Dawson Church

THE PLANTPLUS DIET SOLUTION: Personalized Nutrition for Life, by Joan Borysenko, Ph.D.

RADICAL HOPE: 10 Key Healing Factors from Exceptional Survivors of Cancer & Other Diseases, by Kelly Turner, Ph.D.

All of the above are available at your local bookstore,
or may be ordered by contacting Hay House (see next page).

***

We hope you enjoyed this Hay House book. If you'd like to receive our online catalog featuring additional information on Hay House books and products, or if you'd like to find out more about the Hay Foundation, please contact:

Hay House, Inc., P.O. Box 5100, Carlsbad, CA 92018-5100
(760) 431-7695 or (800) 654-5126
(760) 431-6948 (fax) or (800) 650-5115 (fax)
www.hayhouse.com® • www.hayfoundation.org

———

Published in Australia by: Hay House Australia Pty. Ltd.,
18/36 Ralph St., Alexandria NSW 2015
Phone: 612-9669-4299 • *Fax:* 612-9669-4144
www.hayhouse.com.au

Published in the United Kingdom by: Hay House UK, Ltd.,
The Sixth Floor, Watson House, 54 Baker Street, London W1U 7BU
Phone: +44 (0)20 3927 7290 • *Fax:* +44 (0)20 3927 7291
www.hayhouse.co.uk

Published in India by: Hay House Publishers India,
Muskaan Complex, Plot No. 3, B-2, Vasant Kunj, New Delhi 110 070
Phone: 91-11-4176-1620 • *Fax:* 91-11-4176-1630
www.hayhouse.co.in

———

Access New Knowledge.
Anytime. Anywhere.

Learn and evolve at your own pace
with the world's leading experts.

www.hayhouseU.com

Free e-newsletters from Hay House, the Ultimate Resource for Inspiration

Be the first to know about Hay House's free downloads, special offers, giveaways, contests, and more!

 Get exclusive excerpts from our latest releases and videos from *Hay House Present Moments*.

 Our *Digital Products Newsletter* is the perfect way to stay up-to-date on our latest discounted eBooks, featured mobile apps, and Live Online and On Demand events.

 Learn with real benefits! *HayHouseU.com* is your source for the most innovative online courses from the world's leading personal growth experts. Be the first to know about new online courses and to receive exclusive discounts.

 Enjoy uplifting personal stories, how-to articles, and healing advice, along with videos and empowering quotes, within *Heal Your Life*.

Sign Up Now!

Get inspired, educate yourself, get a complimentary gift, and share the wisdom!

Visit www.hayhouse.com/newsletters to sign up today!

MEDITATE.
VISUALIZE.
LEARN.

Get the **Empower** *You*
Unlimited Audio *Mobile App*

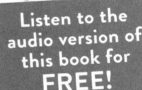

Get unlimited access to the entire Hay House audio library!

You'll get:

- 500+ inspiring and life-changing **audiobooks**

- 200+ ad-free **guided meditations** for sleep, healing, relaxation, spiritual connection, and more

- Hundreds of audios **under 20 minutes** to easily fit into your day

- **Exclusive content** *only* for subscribers

- **New audios** added every week

- No credits, **no limits**

Listen to the audio version of this book for **FREE!**

 ★★★★★ **I ADORE this app.** I use it almost every day. Such a blessing. – Aya Lucy Rose

Scan me with your phone camera!

HAY HOUSE

TRY FOR FREE!
Go to: hayhouse.com/listen-free